Fuel for Thought

Also by Renee McGregor
Training Food
Fast Fuel Food for Running Success
Fast Fuel Food for Triathlon Success
Orthorexia
More Fuel You

Fuel for Thought

A PRACTICAL GUIDE
TO FUELLING FOR
YOUR ADVENTURES

 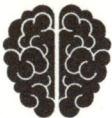 

RENEE McGREGOR

Vertebrate Publishing, Sheffield
www.adventurebooks.com

Fuel for Thought

RENEE McGREGOR

First published in 2025 by Vertebrate Publishing.

Vertebrate Publishing
Omega Court, 352 Cemetery Road, Sheffield S11 8FT, United Kingdom.
www.adventurebooks.com

Copyright © Renee McGregor 2025.
Foreword copyright © Jenny Tough 2025.

Renee McGregor has asserted her rights under the Copyright, Designs and Patents Act 1988 to be identified as author of this work.

This book is a work of non-fiction. The author has stated to the publishers that, except in such minor respects not affecting the substantial accuracy of the work, the contents of the book are true.

A CIP catalogue record for this book is available from the British Library.

ISBN: 978-1-83981-237-8 (Paperback)
ISBN: 978-1-83981-238-5 (Ebook)
ISBN: 978-1-83981-239-2 (Audiobook)

10 9 8 7 6 5 4 3 2 1

All rights reserved. No part of this work covered by the copyright herein may be reproduced or used in any form or by any means – graphic, electronic, or mechanised, including photocopying, recording, taping or information storage and retrieval systems – without the written permission of the publisher.

Every effort has been made to obtain the necessary permissions with reference to copyright material, both illustrative and quoted. We apologise for any omissions in this respect and will be pleased to make the appropriate acknowledgements in any future edition.

Edited by Emma Lockley.
Cover design and layout by Jane Beagley, Vertebrate Publishing;
interior design based on an original design by Geoff Borin, www.geoffborinbooks.com

Vertebrate Publishing is committed to printing on paper from sustainable sources.

Printed and bound in Great Britain by Clays Ltd, Elcograf S.p.A.

For everyone who wants to
find peace with food and exercise

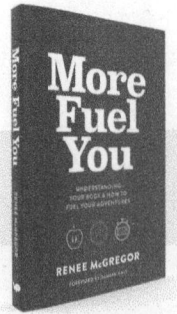 

For more information about *More Fuel You*, visit:
www.adventurebooks.com/more-fuel-you

CONTENTS

FOREWORD by Jenny Tough IX

INTRODUCTION XIII

PART 1: An individual approach 1

  CHAPTER 1: **How it started** 3

  CHAPTER 2: **What kind of runner are you?** 14
    Training age 19
    Why do we find it so difficult to stop? 21
    Knowing when and what to race 22
    What makes someone professional? 23
    The role of stress 27
    When is it time to get a coach? 28
    Is there ever a place for running apps? 30

  CHAPTER 3: **Let's talk about sports nutrition** 33
    Do we all need to worry about obesity? 35
    How do I know if nutrition messages are relevant to me? 36
    Popularity and notoriety 37
    How can we achieve balance? 40
    Can we lose weight while we are exercising? 41
    Does fitness/athleticism have a look? 42
    Is it ever acceptable to lose weight for running performance? 42
    So what and how should you eat? 44
    Beliefs, societal pressures and ideals 45
    My story 47
    Final word 49

PART 2: Putting it into practice 51

  CHAPTER 4: **The store cupboard** 53
    Carbohydrates 53
    Fruit and vegetables 55
    Proteins 56

  Fat 59
  Vitamins and minerals 59
  The gut microbiome 66
  Ergogenic aids 67

CHAPTER 5: **An A to Z of foods** 75

CHAPTER 6: **The kitchen** 96
  The importance of glycogen 96
  Carbohydrate loading 101
  Fuelling your training 102
  Eating on the move 114

CHAPTER 7: **Top tips and example menus** 119
  Top tips 119
  Example day menus 125
  Final word on fuelling for training 129

PART 3: **Humans are not textbooks** 133

 CHAPTER 8: **False refuges and how they hinder us** 135
  Limiting beliefs and dysfunctional behaviours 137
  Understanding dysfunctional behaviours 140
  REDs and low energy availability 141
  Looking after our hormonal health 148
  Exercise dependency 155
  Body image 157
  What do medics need to know? 158
  What's wrong with me? 162

 CHAPTER 9: **Running for life** 165

REFERENCES 169

ACKNOWLEDGEMENTS 173

ABOUT THE AUTHOR 174

FOREWORD

I've been running for twenty years now, starting as a teenager angry at my body, evolving into a marathoner pursuing time goals, and growing into an adventure-chasing trail and ultrarunner. I've naturally been through highs and lows with my sport, my body and the eternal pursuit of trying to be 'better'. Running has taken me around the world and given me a community and friendship circle that is incredibly dear to me. Running saves me from myself and connects me with the beautiful natural world I get to run through. But it can also leave me frustrated – when my body doesn't look like the ultrarunners I see in magazines, when my performance plateaus or even recedes. By the time I met Renee McGregor, I'm sure I had already tried nearly every type of 'diet' that made the rounds in the running world, always hoping that this would be the promised magic recipe to morph my body into the (impossible) standards imposed on female athletes.

When a doctor informed me that I had an eating disorder, I was in disbelief. I had been 'eating healthily' my entire adult life. Carefully avoiding Bad Foods, loading up on Good Foods. I followed sound nutritional advice from trusted authors and athletes who backed up their claims with (supposed) science and results. I hadn't had normal menstrual function in over a decade, but I had been reassured by doctors that this was totally normal for my level of exercise. Besides, I had just won a major ultra race and was maintaining a high level of exercise – only, I had admittedly been slowing down a lot and suffering with debilitating fatigue and difficulty recovering. I had only called the doctor hoping she would offer some bloodwork and tell me I needed an extra macronutrient supplement, or something like that. I didn't expect her to say that I simply wasn't eating enough – and had some profound anxiety around food.

My weight has troubled me since I can remember. It made no sense to me that I might not be eating enough – if I wasn't getting enough, then why wasn't I losing weight? I was losing my hair, so why not my belly?

Recovering from REDs was harder than any ultra I've trained for. It required an entire rewiring of my brain around food. I had to significantly increase my intake and start to let food types back into my diet – or at least learn not to have a panic attack around them. I had to become aware of just how much of my daily thoughts revolved around food and my body composition, and try to turn down the dial on those thoughts.

The entire time, I felt like an outlier, and I still do. A quick scroll through endurance sports-themed social media feeds, magazines, book titles or podcasts, and it seems like nearly everyone is still tossing out the same messages that got me so ill in the first place.

'This one simple trick will help you lose weight'
'How you're sabotaging your fat loss with this ingredient'
'Eat this, not that'
'The secret to losing weight fast'
'Get to racing weight in eight days'
'New way to lose weight, proven by science'

On and on, these tricks and hacks to 'optimising' your body are bombarding athletes, amateur and pro alike. Trendy headlines and beautiful influencers lure us to the magical solution they claim to have found – but wait a few years and a new trend will come along. The goalposts keep moving and we keep buying into a system (the diet industry) designed to fail. They come from all sources on all platforms.

Except for my lovely friend Renee. In the years since her first book, she has stayed consistent in her messaging – I've never seen her adopt a trend, a quick-fix, a *diet*, or debase her years of clinical knowledge in any way to sell more copies or get more followers. She knows what works, what is true, and she is unwavering in spreading that knowledge.

And that's how the penny dropped for me in 'nutritional advice' content. *Everyone* is trying to sell something. Before deciding who to listen to, figure out first what they want to sell. Popular dieting programmes want you to fail so you come back and spend more money. Fad diet authors get huge fame in a short amount of time and sell lots of copies. Magazines and online resources need exciting headlines to grab your attention. They do not need your long-term success. They are simply running a business in a multi-billion-dollar industry.

Combine the capitalist machine pushing these influencers and authors to sell products fast with the often-unrealistic image of athletes' bodies, and you find yourself in a storm of noise with few voices you can trust.

But Renee doesn't want quick fame – she simply wants fewer athletes having GP appointments like the one I had. In my years of recovery, I find myself consistently going back to her books – that I've already read dozens of times – to remind myself what is *true*. When it feels like most runners I know are engaging in harmful practices, largely spurred on by damaging messaging around what a runner's body 'should look like', or confused narratives around 'wellness', I can find myself starting to get confused again. So I go back to Renee. Her expert advice (and I mean truly *expert* – like university-educated, clinical practitioner kind of expert), sensible approach to food for real humans with real lives, and gentle guidance for athletes to find true health and improved performance is my calm in the storm.

In this book, she gently guides us through the truth of how our bodies work when we do sport (and recover!), and how we can meet its needs and feel our very best. Renee opens up about her own relationship with self-image, being a busy working mum, and striving for her own running and adventure goals – and how she manages to balance it all in the real world. She offers gentle guidance, not strict *rules* that you must adhere to. After reading this book, you will feel empowered with a better understanding of what your unique body needs in your unique life to train for your own athletic goals. And, hopefully, you will come away with a better relationship with food.

She even makes a case for ice cream, and I think we can all agree that's very important.

It's hard being a female athlete, especially not having a conforming body type. I still get worried and can be led off the path from time to time, but Renee will always turn to me and say, 'Your body is the least interesting thing about you.'

Jenny Tough

INTRODUCTION

'Foodie adventures are the best adventures', so the quote goes, yet why does it feel like we live in a world where we deny ourselves the pure pleasure of eating?

If you have picked up this book, chances are you have been caught up in all the noise and are looking for a trustworthy voice on not only how to fuel your running adventures but also how to rebuild your trust and relationship with both running and food.

If we strip things back to basics, food should be really simple. It is purely a means by which we nourish our bodies, providing it with the nutrients and fuel we need in order to live, perform and interact with others. And yet, in over two decades of working in this speciality known as nutrition, never before have I seen eating and food become so complicated, confusing and polarised.

Everyone has an opinion, and of course they are entitled to that opinion. But as someone who gets to work with people day in, day out on their nutritional needs, what I hear time and time again is 'I need to get it right!' and this seems to be more important and valuable than the actual joy of eating.

The cost of living is having an impact on all of us with regard to what we can afford to spend on our weekly shop. This is a real issue and a topic I will be addressing later in this book, but from the conversations I am having in the clinic, it goes deeper than just financial constraints. It appears that food is no longer a personal preference. In fact, I would go as far as saying that there is almost shame in choosing food that we want and enjoy. Instead, food choice has become a behaviour influenced by the external world, which then derails us from listening to our internal cues. And it's not just restricted to food. The advent of social media means that we now have access to information 24/7, but no real way of filtering whether this information is appropriate, credible or, more importantly, relevant to us.

If someone says 'running is my job', be wary. Anyone can run, or at least give it a go. Then there are those of us who gain huge enjoyment from it, are prepared to put the hard work in and actually get pretty decent results. I put myself in this camp, but I definitely don't see running as my job and I also know that I am not among the few per cent of individuals who are genetically gifted and have physiological talent that elevates them to professional level.

Professional athletes – and I'm not just talking about the Olympic and Paralympic pathway; I'm talking about athletes who get paid to run because of their ability – can absolutely own 'running is my job'. I have the privilege of working with many of these individuals, and they are very different from the many individuals who from here I am going to call 'run-fluencers', who have flooded on to social media platforms and gained traction because they are really, really good at creating content and selling. They get media places at races, not places based on their running ability.

You may feel that I am being very harsh. While that is not my intention, I really think it is important to be aware of the difference because these run-fluencers often lack responsibility and appear to have no awareness of training age, periodisation or, more importantly, rest and what it actually means to be a true athlete. While I don't believe it is through malice, there is still a real concern about their inability to be mindful that their content can influence unrealistic ideals about training, nutrition and even body composition. Remember, these individuals get paid for their content and they are bloody brilliant at their job, which is why so many of us get sucked in. I hate to say it, but if you follow their lead, it will end in tears. Believe me, I see it unfold daily.

I guess what I'm trying to say is that it's not really your fault! There are so many unregulated individuals and also professional individuals stepping out of their lane, all trying to sell you a lie. We are only human and we want life to be easy, so if we read a post or watch a video that offers us this potential, why wouldn't we absorb it and take it on board?

But it goes further than that. While we have had all these technical advances, our brain and central nervous system hasn't evolved quite as quickly. So while the majority of us in the Western world no longer face the same threats as our ancestors relating to food scarcity, the lack of safe and appropriate shelter, disease or the fear of being eaten, our nervous systems are still on high alert and constantly responding to threats, albeit more socially driven.

INTRODUCTION

Tara Brach, a psychologist I highly respect, summed it up beautifully when she said that we are living in an era where the inherent message in Western society is 'Do more! Accomplish more! Generate more!' and of course this leads to a constant fear of falling short, not being enough or doing enough, which impacts our behaviours when it comes to both food and running.

As much as I hate this to be true, it really feels like many of us have lost trust in our bodies and, moreover, we have lost trust in understanding and responding to them.

And this is why I am writing this book!

While I don't have the authority to write on all subject matters, I do have a wealth of experience, education and knowledge in the area of sports nutrition, running, hormones and generally how to be happier and healthier in our bodies.

I'm fed up with all the noise and, quite frankly, the bullshit advice that is constantly being spouted out of the internet. I want to put the love and fun back into both eating and moving, but more notably running. That doesn't mean novel ingredients or promoting specialist products that most of us would need to take out a second mortgage to sustain. This book is an opportunity to speak common sense, and to use everyday ingredients to produce simple meals and snacks that even my teenage daughters have approved and will vouch are simple to make on a student budget.

My aim is to create a resource that you can go back to again and again, regardless of your running experience, from absolute beginners to hardened veterans to elite and professional athletes, over all distances and terrains. Whether you just want a recipe idea, want to understand how to fuel and train towards your next run event, or need reminding that not everything on social media is attainable or even realistic, this is the book for you.

The purpose of this book is to help you to navigate your journey and understand how to train appropriately, based on you and your training age. It is to help you stop comparing, be realistic about your expectations and actually get the best out of your running.

Over the course of the book, I will cover how my own journey working with runners and becoming a runner myself has influenced my knowledge and, as in my previous books, I will aim to bring my practice to light with case studies and personal anecdotes. I will explore running in detail, covering different types and distances, but also provide education around where you are in your own journey and when it is time to get some external support and help. There will also be numerous practical tips and suggestions on nutrition and fuelling, and a whole section on some of my go-to, tried-and-tested, budget-friendly recipes.

Enjoy,
R x

PART 1

An individual approach

CHAPTER 1

How it started

Why did I get to write this book?

Yes, I'm a professional. Some would even go as far as calling me a sports nutrition expert. I personally struggle with this definition as I'm not sure we can ever be an expert in anything – there is always more to learn and more we don't know. However, I do have authority on this subject matter as my experience of working in the field of nutrition spans more than two decades.

I have worked with runners of all levels and abilities, across all distances and pretty much every terrain, from parkrun to marathon, 24-hour and multi-stage races. On the track, in deserts, on ice-capped mountains, alpine trails and even an airfield. At major championships, the biggest trail and mountain events of the race calendar, local road races and extreme charity challenges. I have worked in it all and seen every mistake, but I've also worked with individual athletes to help them achieve their goals and reach their potential. I have been part of several academic consensus papers looking at specific recommendations around dysfunctional relationships with food such as orthorexia and REDs (relative energy deficiency in sport), and I've been the clinical advisor on many documentaries related to nutrition, sport, body image and athletes.

But, more than that, I'm a runner. You would think my approach to fuelling and running would be bang on the money, but I'm also human. And, like all other humans, my behaviour can be unpredictable and irrational. Not only have I observed and worked with many athletes and individuals and gained knowledge and insight, but I've made my own mistakes time and time again, and no doubt I'll make them again. Granted, I tend to know what I need in the moment, although this doesn't always mean I can come to my own rescue (more on this later), but without sounding arrogant, I don't really know anyone more qualified to write this book.

I have worked with some of the best runners the UK has been blessed with, but if you had asked me as a youngster what my future career ambitions were, nutrition was not one of them. In fact, my favourite subject at school was always English. Maybe this had more to do with the amazing and patient teachers I had, but I loved getting lost in words. That is not to say it came easy. I was born in the UK into a Punjabi Sikh family, and until I went to school, Punjabi was the only language I was fluent in. When I started reception at the age of four, the school advised my parents to speak to me in English at home too so that I would find school easier. Let's just say that school was never easy. I never really fitted in and I was never truly accepted. At secondary school, I spent most of my free time either playing sports or hiding in the library.

You get the picture – I was a pretty quiet, introverted individual and, while people find this hard to believe, I still am. I do a lot of public speaking with my job, but this massively drains my social battery and I often need a full day of quiet, usually hiding in the hills or resting on the sofa with my dogs, to recover. Ewen, my partner, jokes that we should call our house The Hermitage because I really do like to be a hermit, and generally like my own company or the company of a few trusted others.

But I digress ...

While English was my first love, it was not a subject I took at A level. My parents were strict and favoured science. I think I always knew that I wouldn't have much choice when it came to A levels, so I dutifully did maths, biology and chemistry and then applied to university to do biochemistry. I honestly had no clue what I wanted to do at that stage, but my teenage experience of an eating disorder had definitely influenced my interest in the human body. How it all worked. What happened at a cellular level in our bodies. How these intricate chemical reactions that made us human all worked together, and how we had such a big part to play in how well our bodies worked for us.

Three years later, I graduated from Nottingham University with a degree in nutritional biochemistry, which led me to my postgraduate degree in dietetics. This time, I packed my bags and headed to Glasgow. Those two years still stand out in my memory as being some of the best years of my life. My only regret is that I wish twenty-one-year-old Renee had appreciated the proximity to the big hills and mountains and made the most of her time in those, but at that stage in life, my priorities were clubbing, boys and becoming a registered dietitian.

My career started two years later as I began my first role as an entry-level dietitian at St George's Hospital, Tooting, a large London teaching hospital. You are pretty much thrown in at the deep end, with an average caseload of eight to ten wards to look after across a number of clinical specialties, ranging from geriatrics to renal, gastroenterology and outpatient clinics. I had three other clinical roles during my time as an NHS dietitian, each time moving on to a more senior level and becoming more and more specialist. My last role was as a paediatric dietitian specialising in adolescent eating disorders.

My eleven years in the NHS were not only critical but also truly imperative for my growth as a practitioner. They taught me so many important skills and knowledge, but also the most important lesson: 'humans are *not* textbooks'. To this day, this is relevant and I think it is why I get good engagement from the individuals I work with, and is also what makes me different from others.

Don't get me wrong – as any clinician will tell you, evidence-based practice is central to the work you do. However, while scientific theory is important, this doesn't mean that it aligns with someone who is living, breathing and has a mind of their own which can often be influenced by external sources.

Scientific studies tend to be one-dimensional, by which I mean that they are there to test or disprove a hypothesis. However, humans are three-dimensional, and much more than just a simple hypothesis test. So, while academic research may state that if someone does X, Y may happen, this does not take into account anything else that may be going on for that person, or even how physiology, biochemistry and endocrinology may be impacted by or impact a particular intervention.

Presently, for example, one of the big trends in the nutrition sphere is glucose monitoring and there is a lot of scaremongering around the words 'glucose spike'. However, in the context of humans, our blood glucose is impacted by many other influences, such as physical activity, hormones, stress, dehydration and illness. Even if we eat the same foods day after day, our blood sugars will not remain static; they will still fluctuate depending on these potential factors. But even more relevant and important is that, firstly, it is normal for our blood glucose to be out of the recommended range for some of the day without any adverse consequences to health; and secondly, there are times when we actually want to create a glucose spike. After exercise, when we want to replenish our muscles as quickly as possible, taking on fuel such as chocolate milk creates a spike in glucose, which in turn increases insulin levels, which actually helps to draw nutrition back into the body to help repair and replenish it.

Having that deep understanding of how the human body works, appreciating how to critically appraise a scientific study and then working out how to apply it in real-life scenarios is definitely a forte of mine, and one that not everyone has. This is why I always say that you can't beat hands-on experience, actually working in a field. You might have an amazing mind and be incredibly knowledgeable, but you have to know how to apply this in real life. It is something that I have found instrumental, especially when working at big championships like the 24-hour worlds or crewing at a major race like UTMB. The ability to think on my feet and come up with an immediate solution for the athlete I am working with is fundamental to their performance in that given moment.

It's also the big difference between me and the many health professionals who have become digital practitioners – that is, they provide professional advice online. These individuals are a new generation of health practitioners who absolutely have the professional qualifications and title, but this role comes second to creating content. They have built a huge following, due to savvy technology skills and theoretical knowledge, but have never actually worked with individuals (no, answering DMs doesn't count) or in the field they have qualified in. I will discuss this further in later chapters when looking at nutritional requirements and the need for a more nuanced approach.

I left the NHS in 2010 and enrolled on my third degree, this time in applied sports nutrition. I also did fitness instructor qualifications, juggling these with full-time motherhood and some private clinical dietetic work. This is also when I became much more involved in my local running club and started training more specifically for the marathon distance.

I never ran as a child. While I was very sporty, I was terrible at athletics and my main sports were hockey, netball and rounders. I swam as a younger child until I was twelve, when it started to become a bit too much of a commitment alongside schoolwork. I also loved dancing and I have numerous medals and trophies from all the dance competitions I entered with my club. This came to a stop when I was sixteen due to the need to focus on my studies. So you could say that movement in general has always been pretty central to my daily life.

In my early twenties, when I was living and working in London, I started running with a friend a few times a week. We never did more than five miles and the intention was purely to keep fit and decompress from work, which was often intense and stressful. It only lasted a couple of years at this stage.

In January 2003, I gave birth to my first daughter. We were living on a boat in the Docklands and I witnessed Paula Radcliffe get her world-record time at the London Marathon. As I stood there with my ten-week-old baby in my arms, a switch went off: could I run a marathon?

It was actually almost three years later, when I was twenty-nine and my second daughter was eleven months old, that I decided to give running another go. We were still living on a boat but had moved out of London to Bath. We had a lovely mooring on the River Avon and it was the perfect location to run.

My first run there was ten minutes. I was still breastfeeding, had basically just been pushing a buggy for long walks and opening locks as my main form of exercise for the previous three years, and all I wanted was a little break from the boat and being a mum. I loved it – the feeling of moving my body freely again and being out in nature but also on my own, in my own thoughts. I felt like me.

Over the following months, I slowly built this up. I ran three times a week and never for more than an hour, but it was something for me and that was all. It made me happy. It was about five years later that I entered a local race and won. It was very low key and I think I surprised everyone. After the race, the gym owner, who was also the race director, encouraged me to join the local running club so that I could race for them.

Joining the club had many benefits. I met so many like-minded individuals and it was great to finally feel part of a collective, in a space where I felt accepted. While my time in this club was relatively short-lived, it did pave the way for my love of the running community and I am so grateful to this day. I have met some of my closest friends through running, as well as my partner. Running helps to demonstrate who I am. It's the most 'me' I feel – exploring trails, helping me to inner strength and peace. It empowers me to believe that I am enough, regardless of whether I fail or succeed.

Running has led me to many adventures and fun opportunities over the last twenty years. After being a young girl who was bullied and assaulted for the colour of her skin, I found a home and a place where I feel I finally belong in the running community. It also drives my passion and work as a trustee for Black Trail Runners to encourage more accessibility and opportunity for those from minority groups to take up running. But it also means that I get it. I understand the mentality; I appreciate the disappointments and pitfalls. I have tricks up my sleeve that I have learnt – things I have trialled and found to be useful which I can then use with those I work with. When a runner, regardless of level, talks to me about some of their concerns, or has a nutrition question where there is no answer on Google, I can usually come up with a solution. I guess that's why I have been so fortunate to work both with high-performing runners, particularly in the ultra-distance and mountain running space, and also with those who just love running. I am knowledgeable and yet relatable.

Like most people, my running started with a focus on the road. Being part of the club was great for my social connection, but it also fed into my obsessive, perfectionist side. As a teenager, I had an episode of anorexia. Years later, when I was a mum to two still relatively young children and working part-time, the running club gave me an opportunity to do something for me, but it also provided a competitive environment that created the perfect storm for some dysfunctional behaviours to form and old beliefs to return. I became a little obsessive, and I can see now that it wasn't healthy. I guess you could say that I was trying to attain my worth and sense of identity through my running. This is something I see in so many of the individuals I work with now and I will go into more detail about this later in this book. I became fixated on doing more, getting faster and always trying to beat my times, to the point where I actually started to fall out of love with running.

After running three marathons – London twice and Manchester once – and getting the same time at all three (3:17 if you need to know!), it felt like the right time to leave the club, hang up my road-running shoes and turn my attention to trails, mountains and ultra distance. To start with, this was a really good move for me. It took the pressure off; I was no longer a slave to my watch. Instead, I loved the long social miles with friends and started to see races as an opportunity to explore new parts of the UK and also travel abroad.

Joining the running club in Bath also helped to pave the way for my future career in sports nutrition. It was around this time when I enrolled on my third degree. I was getting asked a lot of questions about nutrition and running by my peers, and while I had some basic knowledge and understanding, I wasn't technically qualified in sports nutrition. I appreciate that this is not something that stops many individuals stepping into areas they are not qualified in, but I have a very strong work ethic and moral compass. If I am going to provide nutrition advice in a particular area, then I want to be informed.

It wasn't long after completing my postgraduate degree in applied sports nutrition that the opportunity arose for me to work with the GB rhythmic gymnastics team, who had a wildcard qualification to the 2012 London Olympics. You could say I was pretty much thrown in at the deep end, but wow, what an experience that was! I was so grateful for my previous clinic knowledge. Combining this with my newly acquired sports nutrition qualification really helped to keep those gymnasts safe. The performance world is brutal both for athletes and for those working in it, and there is so much pressure. This is not something I particularly agree with, and it is something I have spoken openly about. With the focus always being on performance, and funding being allocated by medals and achievement, both the physical and mental health of the athletes is overlooked in a lot of instances. Although policies and protocols are always being put in place, they often feel like a box-ticking exercise rather than something that truly safeguards athletes. Things are slowly changing, but only because many athletes have come forward and spoken about their own experiences.

London 2012 opened the door for me. Over the following years, I had the opportunity to work with a vast diversity of athletes and sports, from free diving to England hockey and netball players, eventually leading to the roles of both sports science lead and sports dietitian for the GB wheelchair fencing and wheelchair basketball teams that went to Rio 2016. Heading out to the Paralympic Games in 2016 was one of the most amazing experiences and learning opportunities of my career – there are no words really. It was amazing, exhausting, exhilarating and stressful, all at the same time. The planning, lead-up and then being at a major championships teaches you a unique skill set, and I have been able to transfer this to other roles since, including setting up my own consultancy and clinic. We came back from that Games with a silver and bronze medal for the teams I was involved with.

On paper, it would seem that I had it all as far as my career was concerned. When I was studying for the sports nutrition qualification, my ultimate role was working in high-performance sport and I had achieved this in the first five years of my career in sport. And yet, something didn't feel right. It was eating away at me (sorry, bad pun!). Was this my familiar perfectionist narrative of 'not good enough', or was something more complicated going on?

The longer I worked in sport, the more I became aware of the fine line all athletes teetered on between health and performance. It didn't seem to really matter what sports I worked in, a clear theme was coming through. By 2014 I started to be approached by many high-performance athletes looking for support with what is now known as REDs (see chapter 8) but at that point didn't really have a clear definition. It was known as the 'female athlete triad', which excluded men, and yet I was seeing both genders, mainly across endurance sports such as cycling, running and triathlon. In reality, I was working with individuals who had a dysfunctional relationship with food and exercise, and who couldn't get specialist support from their national governing bodies. It was my previous clinical experience in eating disorders, combined with my knowledge in sports nutrition, that created the bridge for these individuals who were being overlooked by both the clinical and sporting worlds. This became my niche, and by the time an IOC consensus paper came out about REDs in 2016, I had already made so many of the connections between low energy availability, poor health and poor performance. In fact, reading and understanding the psychological, hormonal and physiological connections helped me to appreciate that I too, completely unintentionally, had fallen into this condition we now know as REDs.

My move into trail and mountain running had gone well. I loved it and found that running beyond 26.2 miles was actually my forte. However, even though I was working in the field of sports nutrition, I hugely underestimated how much fuel I needed to keep all parts of my life going – as a mother, runner and sports dietitian. In 2015 I hit a bit of a brick wall with my running. I literally went from racing fifty-kilometre, fifty-mile and multi-day events to crawling overnight. Well, that is what it felt like to me. I genuinely had no idea what had happened, but as someone who had been pretty strong at running up hills, I was having to walk in order to catch my breath. I felt absolutely terrible.

My initial reaction was that I must be deficient in something. I had all my bloods done and everything came back normal, even for someone who is physically active. I was then tested for running-induced asthma, but inhalers made no difference to how running felt. Eventually, my GP ordered a CT scan of my lungs. This is definitely not the call you want to get on a Friday afternoon.

'Excuse me, Mrs McGregor, but we have had the results of your CT back and we have found some significant shadowing which suggests changes within your lungs. We would like you to come in next week to talk to us.'

I remember that call so well. It was an agonising weekend where I was really trying not to panic. Eventually, when I got to see my GP, she told me that they thought I had interstitial lung disease but they would need to do a bronchoscopy and take biopsies to get complete clarity.

According to the American Lung Association, interstitial lung disease (ILD) is 'an umbrella term used for a large group of diseases that cause scarring (fibrosis) of the lungs. The scarring causes stiffness in the lungs which makes it difficult to breathe and get oxygen to the bloodstream. Lung damage from ILDs is often irreversible and gets worse over time.'

A few weeks later, I was sitting in the respiratory consultant's office, waiting to hear what was going on. I was diagnosed with sarcoidosis, an autoimmune lung disease. There had been significant scarring on my lungs, which is why I was struggling to breathe when I was running. It was very unusual, particularly for a woman from Indian origin, there was no real cure, and while some people will see a reversal after two years, for others the scarring is permanent damage that they will have to live with. While the consultant didn't say I couldn't run, she did say that I would need to run according to my symptoms and, unless the scarring reversed, it was unlikely that I would ever get back to my previous form.

I was devastated because at that moment in time I was unable to run. Over the following eighteen months, my condition got worse and worse. In 2017, post-divorce, I had moved into a little cottage over three floors in Bradford-on-Avon, and I was out of breath just going up and down the stairs. I was exhausted. This is something no one really tells you about so many autoimmune conditions: the extreme fatigue. I felt so awful, and yet if you'd looked at me, you wouldn't have known there was anything wrong.

I remember trying to manage my work at this stage, and it was so hard. There were days when I was literally dragging myself to work. I had turned my attention to yoga and had come to really enjoy it, but I still missed running. In December of that year, I once again sat in the consultant's office. My symptoms had been getting worse, she had repeated the tests and CT, and it wasn't good news. It was clear that my condition was permanent and my lung function had dropped to 73%, where it remains to this day. She was talking about steroid treatment and all I remember thinking was, *How has this happened?*

I asked for the Christmas break to think about everything and said I would come back to her in the new year with my thoughts. Weirdly, my work with athletes and all the reading I had been doing about helping them with REDs brought a new understanding to my own condition. REDs is a multi-system condition, and one of the areas that is rarely talked about is the impact it has on immune health.

By that stage, I had actually taken a step back from my work with Olympic and Paralympic sports and my consultancy was in full swing. I was very busy and had very much become the go-to person for athletes of any age, any sport and any level to get help with REDs, dysfunctional relationships with food and exercise, and hormonal health. Ultimately, that little niggle I had had about things not feeling right on my return from Rio had grown. I knew that, for me, the health of an athlete was way more important than the performance; but I also knew that without their health, athletes can't perform. While it was not an easy decision to make, I knew working in high-performance sport didn't align with my values and it was making me unhappy, regardless of how the job appeared. In fact, when I left, I got told that I cared too much, but that was enough of a reason for me to know I had made the right decision. And when one door closes, others open. Without this, I probably wouldn't be where I am today, working with the range of athletes I do, being the Nutrition Lead at two of the main ballet companies in the UK (English and Scottish), supporting both their health and performance needs, and in some cases providing them with a lifeline back into performance sport and dance.

They always say that you can never see what is going on right under your nose, and while I had an inkling that maybe my running had contributed to my sarcoidosis diagnosis, it wasn't something I understood or really wanted to believe. Although no medical practitioner has directly said this, bearing in mind the lack of crossover between the clinical and sports world, I am a clinician and practitioner in my own right, and on reflection it has become clear to me that I just overloaded my nervous system (that is the central nervous system – the brain and spinal cord – and the peripheral nervous system). In those previous twenty-four months, I had raced five ultra-distance events, including a multi-day race at high altitude in Nepal; I had been working full-time in a stressful environment, due to preparations for the 2016 Paralympics; I was a full-time mum to two daughters aged eleven and thirteen; my marriage was going through a really rocky patch; I was training hard, often waking up super early to get my training done in a fasted state; and I was probably in low energy availability 50% of the time, albeit completely unintentionally. In fact, this is everything I try to help the individuals I work with to manage now. So not only do I understand the science and physiology behind under-recovery, fasted training and the consequences of layer upon layer upon layer of stress on the body, but I have also got the T-shirt. I guess this is why I have empathy and compassion but also a direct response to all those I work with. The aim is to always prevent a prolonged absence from their sport and moreover to help them become sustainable athletes with longevity.

And what about my sarcoidosis now? Well, I'm sadly one of those individuals where the scarring on my lungs is permanent and I still only have 73% lung function. At the last CT scan of my lungs in 2023, thankfully there was no further scarring. And I have been back running for a few years now.

I have learnt how to manage my condition, but I want to add the caveat that this is personal to me and everyone who lives with an autoimmune condition has to find their own path. There is definitely a threshold of stress that my body can cope with, and when I tip over this, it is always my immune system that takes the hit. Nowadays, I manage my training load under the watchful eye and support of my coach, Damian Hall, and I manage stress alongside this in order to maintain my status quo and hopefully prevent a further flare-up.

Despite all this, working with Damian has resulted in some of my best performances. In the last few years, I was British trail running champion over the short course (20 kilometres) in my age category, and third female and ninth overall in the Summer Spine Sprint 2022. I have also returned to my beloved Nepal and finished fourth female and eighth overall in the Mustang Trail Race in 2023.

And I guess that brings us up to the present day. As I sit here, looking out of the window as the rain falls over Kendal, my new home and very happy place, with the dogs gently snoring on the sofa behind me, I feel a huge sense of privilege that I get to write this book, hopefully set the record straight on a number of key areas and, most importantly, inform and educate you to help you become the healthiest and most sustainable runner you can be, regardless of how long you have been running, or what level you may or may not compete at.

Let's get started, shall we?

CHAPTER 2

What kind of runner are you?

I often struggle with this question, because from my point of view, anyone who runs is a runner. The key thing here is about appreciating where you are in your journey and, most importantly, your relationship with running.

Running is personal and we all run for different reasons. Let's take me as an example. When I first started running, it really was just to get some space from home and mum life. It was an opportunity to connect with nature, my body and myself. I would run for twenty to forty minutes up to three times a week, depending on what life allowed. I built up really slowly and had been running for several years before I considered my first marathon, let alone the move into ultra distance. And let's not forget, I had been a super-active child, swimming six days a week for many years, dancing, and playing hockey and netball. Even after university, I continued to play hockey and joined a gym around the same time as I got my first job as a dietitian in London.

Over time, this has changed. I would now describe myself as an experienced runner and I have been running for over twenty years. I run around five times a week and I also ensure appropriate behaviours such as resistance training, sufficient fuelling and rest to prevent injury.

I would say I'm fairly competitive but definitely not professional. I tend to choose one or two main goals a year and follow a training plan that helps me to arrive at these goals as prepared as I can be. I started with road running, but I am most definitely a trail, mountain and fell runner now. However, I am also very aware and mindful that running is my hobby, and so training, while important to me, is not always a priority. There are also several months within the year where I don't follow a fixed plan and the only real outcome for my running is participation, social connection, mental health and my love of the great outdoors. However, in my experience, not everyone has a healthy relationship with running.

Running is big business at the moment. While road running has long been established, the number of people participating in trail, ultra-distance and extreme running challenges has risen exponentially in the last few years. While I welcome the growth in participation in running, I definitely have some concerns around those with little previous running or athletic experience moving straight into long-distance events. We have seen a huge rise in run-fluencers, some of whom get paid to create content to promote brands, races and events, but a lot of whom don't. One of the concerns here is that as content creation is their job, they are combining their training (and racing) hours with their work, leading to unrealistic ideals and expectations for those of us who are trying to fit training around a more traditional 9–5 job or even shift work.

While run-fluencers' motivation to document their running journey may be innocent, their lack of knowledge and qualifications does mean that their content is at times irresponsible. From sharing 'what I eat in a day' videos to giving details about specific runs and paces, this all feeds into the psyche of others and can cause real problems. Regardless of how big their following, remember that a lot of them will be providing information based on $n=1$ (a sample size of one – that is, their own experience), not scientific papers or, even more importantly, actually working in the field. While I'm all for individuals documenting their own progress, is this something that needs to be shared with everyone else?

This is why identifying where you are on your running journey really does matter, so that you can make appropriate choices about the next steps that are relevant to you, not because a run-fluencer you have chosen to follow is telling you what they are doing next.

I would go as far as questioning that individual's motivation for creating such a post – what are they getting out of it? Is it validation and adoration, or are they promoting something they need you to buy into?

The days are long gone when Instagram was just a place where people

FUEL FOR THOUGHT

TYPE OF RUNNER	NUMBER OF RUNS PER WEEK	TYPE OF RUNS PER WEEK	AIM OF RUNS	POTENTIAL OUTCOME	ADDITIONAL REQUIREMENTS
Social runner	Up to 3 times a week, not necessarily consistently	Easy, steady pace, 30–45 minutes Can be on any terrain	Regular movement Cardiovascular fitness Social connection Mental health Body composition Getting outdoors	Participate in parkrun	
New runner	Running 3 times a week for 2–3 years	Easy/steady runs but maybe starting to include 1 slightly longer run per week Can be on any terrain	Maintaining fitness Increasing endurance Social connection Mental health Benefits of outdoors	Starting to think about joining a running club Potentially entering a few races	Maybe starting to think about adding some resistance training to support the running Starting to be mindful of fuelling, especially if adding longer runs
Building up	Running 4–5 times a week for 3–5 years	Mixture of runs – some easy, some faster tempo Interval-type sessions 1 long run per week Can be on any terrain	Maintaining fitness Increasing endurance Increasing speed Social connection Mental health Benefits of outdoors	Regularly taking part in races from 10km to marathon distance Potentially thinking of some shorter multi-day events	Definitely adding in resistance training to support running and reduce injury risk Considering nutritional intake, especially ahead of faster and longer sessions Thinking about periodisation of training – maybe working with a coach or a downloaded generic training plan or using a running app for the same reason

Table 2.1: Types of runner

posted their holiday photos for family and friends. Now we use our social media accounts to promote our own personal brands. I include myself in this. In an ideal world, I would not be on social media, but I see Instagram as an opportunity to have an educational platform so that everyone can have access to my knowledge to a certain degree. I am incredibly mindful about how much personal information I put on there, and I never discuss specifics about my

WHAT KIND OF RUNNER ARE YOU?

TYPE OF RUNNER	NUMBER OF RUNS PER WEEK	TYPE OF RUNS PER WEEK	AIM OF RUNS	POTENTIAL OUTCOME	ADDITIONAL REQUIREMENTS
Experienced	Running a minimum of 5 times a week for a minimum of 5 years	Easy runs 1–2 harder runs per week 1 long run per week Can be on any terrain	Maintaining fitness Increasing endurance Increasing speed Social connection Mental health Benefits of outdoors	Regularly taking part in races, building up to ultra distance if that is something they want to do Potentially thinking of some longer multi-day events	Definitely adding in resistance training to support running and reduce injury risk Considering nutritional intake, especially ahead of faster and longer sessions Thinking about periodisation of training – maybe working with a coach
Professional runner	Running a minimum of 5 times a week Potentially coming from a background in sport or activity at a junior or semi-professional level for several years Usually sponsored or running for a team Full-time athlete	Mixed runs with a minimum of 2 hard sessions per week and 1–2 longer runs per week, depending on training cycle Can be on any terrain	Running to compete	Regularly taking part in races, with 1–2 main target races for the year	Working with a wrap-around performance team, usually consisting of coach, sports dietitian, physio, sports psychologist and strength and conditioning Definitely periodising training and ensuring good periods of rest to ensure optimal performance when competing

Table 2.1: Types of runner *(continued)*

training or fuelling. I do of course provide nutritional content, but as much as possible, I keep it generic. And while social media platforms may not have any regulations about who can post what, the Health and Care Professions Council, which is the regulatory body for all allied health professionals in the UK, including dietitians (but not nutritionists), has very strict criteria and codes of conduct about what we can and can't say.

So, back to what type of runner are you?

As I've already pointed out, understanding where you are on your journey means you can make ongoing decisions about your running in an informative manner which will not only support your performance but also reduce injury risk and actually increase your longevity in the sport.

While table 2.1 (previous pages) is by no means definitive, I wanted to create something to help people identify where they are and see the steps to healthy progression, if that is what they want to do. In my clinic, especially in recent years and particularly since Covid, I have seen far too many individuals literally go from running three times a week for maybe thirty to forty-five minutes to keep fit, to suddenly deciding six months later they are going to run their first ultramarathon. While they can probably do it with grit and determination, there are a number of reasons why it might not be the right approach. The fact that they have ended up in a clinic consultation with me provides enough information to appreciate why a longer-term outlook is preferred when it comes to running.

I know a lot of you will look at this table and think, *I didn't follow any of this advice!* Maybe some of you will be acutely aware of where you have gone wrong; while others will think, *Well, this is all just rubbish: I have only been running for two years and I've already done two 100-mile races.* Maybe you are lucky, or perhaps you have a long training age (see the next section) behind you that means your body is already accustomed to a high training load. However, I can't stress enough the importance of taking your time to build up your running. There is definitely some leeway in the specific times and distances stated in the table, but as running becomes more and more popular, I have seen many casualties as a result of ignoring this advice.

CASE STUDY

Earlier this year, I started working with a twenty-one-year-old female runner. She had started running about a year and a half earlier during the Covid pandemic. Prior to this, she had been involved in lightweight rowing and had got to the stage where she was invited to trials for a GB place, but she realised that she did not have a healthy relationship with this sport and moved into triathlon. She stopped triathlon training during Covid restrictions when she could no longer go swimming.

On assessment, she reported to me that she had a past history of anorexia nervosa that had started at the age of fourteen, but she had managed to restore her weight and menstruation a couple of years later. She reported that her weight still fluctuated quite a bit and her menstruation had once again stopped. She had not had a period for five years.

She had booked in to see me due to recurrent injuries, including four stress fractures since she had started running. She also told me that she had signed up for a 110-kilometre ultrarun in nine months, having never run above 20 kilometres before.

During our assessment, it was clear that she had made a number of changes to her approach to training and nutrition in the previous six months as a result of appreciating that her stress fractures were most likely related to low hormonal levels, insufficient fuelling and building her volume up too quickly.

We discussed training age and I encouraged her to reconsider the 110-kilometre race and to maybe take racing off the agenda until her menstruation was restored and had been established for a minimum of six months. We also discussed the importance of resistance training and how this can build a strong framework to support running.

One month after our initial session, her menstruation returned. Since then, she has changed her whole approach to training and also takes into consideration stress on her body associated with other areas of her life. She has also been happy to consider racing in a few years' time when she has built up her base, and for now is focusing on resistance training and shorter runs to help future-proof her body.

Training age

The majority of professional athletes have a long training age behind them. Training age is the amount of time an athlete has spent training consistently in a specific physical activity. That would make my training age as a runner twenty years, but if you also add in the years I spent swimming at a relatively competitive level and the years of netball and hockey, my training age is more like thirty-five years, and there is a lot to be said about this. Training age helps to determine the body's ability to withstand load and volume. It's not the only contributing factor – nutrition, rest, genetics and cross-training all have a role to play. However, I am seeing more and more individuals who have jumped straight to the ultra distance. While their bodies may well let them get away with this once, perhaps even twice, the majority end up in my clinic within twelve to eighteen months of starting their running journey, usually with some sort of bone stress or recurrent connective tissue injury.

Coincidentally, while running the Lakeland 50 recently, I got chatting to a fellow runner who happened to follow me on Instagram and had read my previous book, *More Fuel You*. We were discussing running and he told me that he was using the next few years to build up his experience and training age because he was keen to give the Dragon's Back Race a proper go. He had tried previously but was able to see that his lack of running experience meant he wasn't ready for such an extreme challenge. This approach is pretty rare, so it really was refreshing to hear it. For those of you who don't know, the Dragon's Back is a six-day stage race that starts at the top of Wales at Conwy Castle and ends at Cardiff Castle. The days are long, the terrain is technical, especially in the first three days, and the cut-offs are tight. It is definitely not a race to go into without sufficient or appropriate preparation.

Similarly, when you look at most professional athletes, while they may race regularly at smaller events to keep themselves sharp, they tend to only focus on one or two events a year, ensuring a periodised approach to their training throughout the year and significant rest to benefit from that training.

While I have been running for twenty years, I've rarely done more than one or two races a year. A lot of this has to do with appreciating that juggling training for a big event with my job adds a significant amount of stress on my nervous system. I've learnt from my previous experience and I now know I have to manage my overall 'life' load, which includes training, racing, work and home life. However, I am aware that this is not common practice.

CASE STUDY

A couple of years ago, I worked with a twenty-six-year-old male runner. From his history, it was clear that he had always been relatively active, even as a young lad, but he had been running less than a year. He was working in the fitness industry, but had only come to this a few years earlier and it was a big change from his corporate job.

He had a normal BMI (body mass index) of 23. His first event had been a fifty-kilometre ultra-distance race ten months earlier. Since then, he had participated in three further races, all above 100 kilometres. He had presented with a stress reaction, which was confirmed as a full bone stress fracture a few days later.

During our assessment, it was clear that he had been under-fuelling, particularly carbohydrate, which had resulted in a very low testosterone level. His physio confirmed that it was the combination of under-recovery and low testosterone that had left his bone health compromised. In such individuals, weak spots develop within the bones, making them more susceptible to a stress reaction or full-blown stress fracture.

While he rehabbed his stress fracture and restored his testosterone levels, he struggled to take advice from me and his physio regarding the importance of rest and periodisation. Less than a year later, he once again presented with a stress response in the same place.

Why do we find it so difficult to stop?

While these are just a couple of examples, sadly this is becoming a very familiar presentation in my clinic. It is one of the main reasons I really worry about the rise and popularity of running, especially ultrarunning.

Like professional athletes, most runners tend to have certain personality traits. These are not problematic as such, but traits associated with perfectionism, obsessive compulsion, addiction and self-criticism can encourage a more complex relationship with running. If an individual has no self-awareness of these traits or hasn't learnt how to manage them, it puts them at a higher risk of developing a more dysfunctional relationship with running, increasing their risk of injury and illness.

Numerous studies have shown the negative correlation between social media use and self-esteem. Self-esteem refers to feelings of love, respect and trust that a person feels towards themself as a result of knowing themself and evaluating themself realistically, accepting their abilities and strengths as they are and embracing themself.[1]

Self-esteem has a very important place in human life. Many aspects of life impact our self-esteem, but among the most significant are our early experiences with caregivers. The psychologist Tara Brach says, 'Children should be seen; children should be loved for what is seen.'

While many individuals grow up in stable environments that demonstrate unconditional acceptance, many do not, and they often learn to attain worth through achievement. They are accepted for their ability rather than who they are, and this can become an inherent part of their identity. Indeed, many of the individuals I work with in clinic describe themselves as 'the sporty one' in their family, or 'the healthy one' in their friendship groups. This identification often leads to extreme behaviours in an endeavour to feel relevant and worthy.

So, if it is all about our early experience, how does social media fit in?

Social media is available 24/7 and our brains are exposed to a constant influx of information. The more we use it, the more we absorb, and the more the soundbites of information get caught up in our brain chemistry and start to inform us. If our feeds are full of people discussing their training, their nutrition and their racing, we can't help but get caught up in all that noise. This provokes comparison and, while it doesn't affect everyone, it does have a tendency to set up a sense of unworthiness, even in individuals who have grown up with a strong sense of worth. It creates a feeling of falling short in some way. When everyone is always doing something, we can feel uneasy when we are not. This sense of unease and discomfort tends to be the driving force, and a need to somehow 'feel okay' leads to a fixation with running, eating and even our bodies. These all provide a distraction from the real problem: that sense of 'not being good enough' or 'not doing enough'.

With so many events and options available, it is easy to see how so many people feel the need to keep moving forwards. Everyone wants the title of 'most extreme' because they can carry it around like a badge of honour for all of five minutes until they start thinking about what's next.

Knowing when and what to race

As well as appreciating where you are in your running journey, it is also useful to know when to start racing and what type of event your mind and body are ready for. I find the following scale that has been developed by my friends Kirsty Reade and Allie Bailey a really helpful tool and I am very appreciative that they have allowed me to include it. The individual ratings are out of 5, depending on the level of challenge (with 5 being the hardest).

RACE	DRAGON'S BACK RACE	NORTHERN TRAVERSE	LAKELAND 100	THAMES PATH 100
Distance	5	5	4	4
Elevation	5	3	3	1
Surface	5	4	3	1
Navigation	5	5	4	1
Degree of autonomy	4	5	2	2
Lack of sleep	3	5	2	2
TOTAL	27	27	18	11

Table 2.2: The Reade and Bailey scale

What makes someone professional?

It is important to remember that we all have different physiology. Runners who compete in the elite arena often have genetic and physiological traits that give them that extra edge when it comes to performance. In the last twenty years, at least a hundred endurance-related genetic markers have been found to be linked to elite endurance athlete status.[2] While a lot more research is required to understand the full extent of how this influences performance, it does suggest that for some of us, even if we train like demons, we will hit a physiological ceiling limiting our ability and performance outcomes. There is nothing wrong with this and it definitely means that we should consider all the factors necessary to optimise our performances if that is our chosen outcome, but it is also important to have the self-awareness to appreciate where our limits might be.

I've listened to a lot of professional elite-level runners discussing what puts them in that world-class arena. Most put it down to hard work, determination and never giving up. I have no doubt that these characteristics contribute to their success. We all know that athletes and runners tend to have a very determined mindset, but they often overlook the fact that not all of us can achieve what they have done, even if we were put in exactly the same training block and lifestyle. They are definitely gifted. It is a combination of their genetics, physiology, lifestyle, mindset and hard work that gives them that athletic advantage.

Being a professional runner usually means training full-time. To enable this fully, they usually need some sort of funding, which may come from UK Sport if they are on a GB pathway going into an Olympic or Paralympic discipline; or if they are in the trail, fell and mountain running world, they may have a brand sponsor. In both cases, it is important to appreciate that there are different levels even within these funding streams. UK Sport offers payment depending on classification, with those who are more highly ranked receiving more financial support than others. This does mean that some athletes have to find additional sponsorship or must work part-time to support their running and training endeavours. They also can compete to earn money, which is why so many track and field athletes compete at the Diamond League and other similar sportives. Even within branded sponsorship, the levels vary, with top performers being paid an actual wage which is topped up by prize money and bonus payments for prestigious wins. Other brands may support athletes with kit, race entries and travel, but don't necessarily offer a wage. This is very different from a brand ambassador, who still has a role with regard to promoting kit, but don't be fooled into thinking that this makes them a professional athlete. Full disclosure: I am a Montane athlete and, while I perform a role for the brand, namely putting out responsible content around fuelling and running, I do not see myself as a professional athlete. Yes, I do compete, but I do not get paid for my athletic ability.

I spoke to Matt Hickman, marketing director at Montane, about how they choose their athletes and ambassadors. Matt explained that they try to have a Performance Team of individuals who have been chosen on their ability and also those who have a skill set that supports performance. I was chosen for this team through being a voice of authority of nutrition, but had also impressed by results (finishing third lady at the Summer Spine Sprint 2022). They also have a Community Team, who are ambassadors and primarily promote the brand, but they always try to ensure that these people are aligned to brand values to ensure authenticity and responsibility.

In addition, a lot of professional runners surround themselves with a support team. Sometimes when a runner is part of a national governing body, they will be able to access this support via them. In other scenarios, athletes may hand-pick their team. The team will often include a coach, a sports dietitian, a sports psychologist, and a strength and conditioning coach. There will also be an associated medic. Generally, this team works in a multi-disciplinary manner to support the athlete and ensure that they stay well and optimise their performances.

It is important to highlight that professional runners come from very different backgrounds. While the likes of Paula Radcliffe started at a very young age and worked through the ranks, others, particularly in the ultra-distance world, started running a lot later in life. If we take three athletes I work with – Damian Hall, Germain Grangier and Elsey Davis, all of whom have had huge successes in some of the toughest and most notorious mountain and ultra races in the world – their backgrounds are very different.

Damian started his running career in 2011 when he did the Bath Half Marathon. I started to provide support in 2013 when he undertook his first Spine Race. The rest is history, as they say. However, prior to 2011, Damian didn't run. He had played football in his twenties in a semi-professional capacity, but otherwise his route into endurance sport was actually hillwalking. He is an INOV8 athlete and signed up with them in 2015. He still works as a journalist and author, and would describe himself as a semi-professional trail runner. He also supports a lot of causes relating to climate action and is co-founder of The Green Runners and Into Ultra, which provides ultrarunning support to individuals who don't have the finances to take part or purchase kit.

Similarly, Germain started running in 2011. Prior to this, he had a background in alpine skiing as a teenager, and he still participates in skimo (ski mountaineering) during the winter months in preference to running. He then moved into biking and was a very good road cyclist. He was just at the point of going pro when he got an injury in his hip which stopped his progress. At that stage, he had to stop biking and the only thing he could do was run uphill. In 2015 he started working for INOV8 France in their marketing department, but by 2017 he was offered a full-time athlete contract. Since then, he has moved brands and now runs for The North Face.

Elsey comes from a club running background. She started to appreciate that she might be good at this running lark when she did her first sub-three-hour marathon in 2014 uncoached. She then got a coach and started knocking quite big chunks of time off her marathon PB. In 2016 she was called up to represent England, but she was also juggling a full-time role as a junior doctor. She was training before and after twelve-hour shifts and remembers just feeling exhausted and empty. Sadly, she didn't get to run her first selection as it coincided with her first stress fracture. Between 2016 and 2019, she experienced a lot of injuries. She changed coaches in 2018 and also started doing a little bit of work with me. She set her marathon PB of 2:33 at the Valencia Marathon. She was called up again to represent England but got another stress fracture. During Covid, she swapped to trail as she was becoming disheartened by road running and the constant stream of injuries. She also dropped down to working part-time. She took part in the GB trials for the trail team and won, and this opened the door to many more successes, including finishing third at the

Golden Trail Series and a win at the Eiger Ultra Trail race. She signed up with The North Face and decided to go full-time for a year and take a break from her career. Elsey is now back working part-time as a doctor and really enjoys the balance. She told me that she feels working helps her to reduce the pressure and value she was placing on training, and actually makes her a better athlete.

FUN FACTS ABOUT THESE THREE ATHLETES

Damian
- Favourite breakfast: several slices of toast with nut butter topped with banana, and many cups of tea.
- Favourite trail snack: hummus and avocado sandwiches made with white bread.
- Key piece of information he has learnt from working with me: the benefit of eating enough. Appreciating the importance of carbohydrates and also adding protein as an option for fuel during long races.

Germain
- Favourite breakfast: 3–4 slices of bread with butter, 2 scrambled eggs, 1 kiwi with some Skyr and almond butter.
- Favourite pre-run snack: granola.
- Key piece of information he has learnt from working with me: stick to what works and make small tweaks to test, but don't be afraid to go back to what has previously worked well. Shiny, new and exciting is not always the best option.

Elsey
- Favourite breakfast: a big pile of Weetabix with milk and berries, topped with muesli.
- Favourite trail snack: Sesame Snaps.
- Key piece of information she has learnt from working with me: the importance of balance. Appreciating that life stresses can also add to training stress, which was one of the key contributors to her recurrent injuries early on in her running career. Over the years, she has learnt to achieve a more appropriate load, in both life and training.

I want to point out that professional runners are not immune to dysfunctional behaviours, with many falling into the same traps as the rest of us of under-fuelling, under-recovering and not listening to their bodies, which can lead to recurrent injuries and poor performances.

I have been fortunate enough to work with many high-profile runners over the years and it is clear within a few meetings who will have longevity and who will struggle to meet their potential. This is not through lack of hard work, but usually lack of appreciation that their bodies need to be nurtured in a particular way to be successful, just like the rest of us.

The role of stress

Often when we talk about stress, it brings to mind negative connotations, and to a certain extent this is true. Prolonged stress can have negative consequences for the body and increase the risk of physical and mental illness.

In reality, stress is the body's reaction to any change that requires an adjustment or a response. In runners, *some training stress* is required for athletic adaptation and progress. It is also important to note that if there is no stress applied to muscular tissues, a runner's body will simply not adapt to the training. Thus, loading and stressing the tissues is a good thing, provided that the training load does not exceed the body's capacity to adapt.

Running brings about two types of stress: cardiovascular and mechanical. It has been well documented that running causes greater stress on the body than other sports such as cycling or swimming.[3]

Mechanical stress relates to the forces placed on bones, joints and muscles. If the mechanical stress surpasses the body's ability to adapt, the runner is more likely to get injured. Furthermore, a higher mechanical stress without proper recovery will lead to accumulated fatigue in the muscle tissues. Thus, the ability to sustain a fast pace – or even run at all – will be decreased dramatically.

Cardiovascular stress is linked more to the pressure placed on the individual due to the workout. In particular, this can have a big impact on endurance runners. Even if a runner is working at a submaximal intensity of 60–80%, if this is prolonged (over two hours), this combination causes a high level of stress to the runner. Once again, if the individual does not recover or this is not managed well, it can lead to burnout, overtraining, under-recovery and REDs (more on this later), terms which are often used interchangeably.

So, while some stress is necessary, it can become problematic if it is not managed or monitored. What a lot of runners don't appreciate is that the body can't really differentiate between stress from training, particularly cardiovascular stress, and other stresses within the body.

Under-fuelling, being a lower weight than your body genetically wants to be, poor sleep, work and lifestyle stress all put a lot of pressure on the body, in particular the nervous system. When this becomes chronic, the body often gets to a place where it can no longer cope. Ironically, when we notice stress, a lot of us choose to go for a hard or long run, actually adding stress to the system rather than decreasing it.

As I mentioned in the introduction, I'm pretty certain that my own diagnosis of the autoimmune condition sarcoidosis was in response to an overload of stress. My consultant also alluded to this, especially as it came at a time where my marriage was falling apart, I was working in a very pressurised environment preparing for the Rio Paralympics, I was training hard, often in the early morning and often fasted, and my overall physical recovery was poor. While the damage to my lungs is permanent, the other symptoms associated with my sarcoidosis disappeared when I started to take note of and manage all the stresses in my life. I have to monitor all the different plates I spin to ensure that I prevent an active episode occurring again.

When is it time to get a coach?

This brings me nicely on to this section. I am not unique in having to manage many aspects of my life, including my training, to ensure that I don't get sick. This is something I tell most runners I work with because overload can happen to any of us, especially in the current climate where everyone appears to be going at a million miles an hour while constantly being productive and making progress (run-fluencers, I am looking at you!).

One of the things that has helped me is having a coach, although I am not an elite athlete and have never aspired to be one. I understand my physiological limits, I enjoy running and I definitely want to reach my potential. For me, having someone to help plan my training around my work and life keeps me accountable and prevents me from falling back into under-recovery.

I started working with Damian in 2020. We had known each other for a long time and it was actually Damian who asked if I wanted a coach. He said that he saw real potential in me and wanted to help. I was a little taken aback that the great Damian Hall said this to me, someone who had barely been back running for two years since her sarcoidosis diagnosis. To be honest, I was really unsure. While I could see how it might work, I wasn't sure if coaching was for me. I had had a coach in my marathon days and while I did benefit from this, I found the whole process quite stressful, which defeated the object. I found myself trying to work for my coach, rather than my coach working for me, and I came to the conclusion that maybe I was uncoachable because I had so many constraints on my time, like work and being a mum.

I was honest with Damian, but he encouraged me to give it a go. He took time to listen to the demands of my hectic work schedule and my commitments to my girls. He asked and continues to ask me a lot of questions about my health, my sleep and my menstrual cycle, and tailored my training around this. It has felt really supportive and nurturing, and I have got some of my best results in ultra-distance races under his coaching. Even now, as I navigate the perimenopause, he is always happy to listen to my fears but also discuss my energy levels to ensure that running is something that never becomes a stress to me.

So, when is the right time to get a coach, and do you actually need one?

If we refer back to table 2.1 at the start of this chapter, I would say the right time to consider working with a coach is probably once you've been running for a few years and you're starting to think about targeting key races. While I appreciate that it does involve a financial commitment, and the cost of a coach varies a great deal, I still think this is a good investment and I often recommend this to runners I work with instead of a running app (more on this later).

When it comes to choosing a coach, my advice is to talk to a few, work out what you really want from a coach and see who you feel most comfortable with. I would also say, don't be afraid to stop working with one if it doesn't feel right or if their values seem different from yours. Remember that a coach has to work for you, not the other way around!

CASE STUDY

In December 2022, a thirty-four-year-old mum of two children under the age of five came to work with me. She wanted support with her nutrition as she had signed up for the London Marathon and was about to start training. She had previously had a tricky time with her running and several injuries had meant that she had to take a significant amount of time off running, but she had been cross-training during that time.

As we started talking, it became clear that her training volume was very high and her nutritional intake was not sufficient to meet the demands of her training. She was working with a coach, but the more she told me about her training plan, the more concerned I became. It didn't feel like this particular coach appreciated what it meant for her to be a mum to two small children while also juggling her own business and training.

We had a long chat about her goals and she said that she would be interested in talking to other coaches who might be a better fit for her. I put her in touch with one of the coaches I often recommend for being knowledgeable, responsible and available, which was going to be essential to help her manage her load.

She started working with the new coach, who was also a mum, and over the next few months there was a real change in her attitude towards training. She went on to get a marathon PB and since then has also ventured into other types of running, including trail and ultra distance. However, her training load is significantly lower than when I first met her, she is eating much better and her relationship with running has significantly changed for the better.

Is there ever a place for running apps?

While I can totally appreciate the appeal of using a running app – after all, they are much more affordable than a running coach – I would urge caution. Remember that one of the benefits of a coach is the personal interaction. You can speak to them and discuss how you are feeling, and decide on optimal training and appropriate racing.

While running apps provide the convenience of guidance, what many lack is the ability to adjust training according to life and also ability. Many just involve inputting very basic information, choosing a plan (whether that be half marathon, marathon or ultra distance) and then pressing go. There is no consideration of what type of runner you are (see table 2.1), and as we know this can have severe consequences, especially with regard to injury risk.

My advice is to maybe use a running app as a framework but still try to be guided by how you are feeling. If you have a really full-on work week, reduce the intensity so that you are not adding stress or unnecessary pressure to your nervous system. Similarly, if you notice a niggle, stop and ideally get advice from a professional. If you are a female runner and you notice changes to your menstrual cycle, stop and get advice from a professional. If you are a female runner and don't have a menstrual cycle without a valid medical reason, please do not sign up to a running app and instead seek advice from a professional. If you are a male or female runner and on paper are underweight, please speak to a professional before embarking on a training plan with an app. If you are a beginner, where possible choose running apps that take this into consideration and have beginner, intermediate and experienced plan options. Similarly, be mindful of how quickly a plan builds volume and particularly intensity. The 10% rule (in order to stay injury-free, never increase your weekly mileage by more than 10% from one week to the next) is there for a reason, but it is important for you to be aware of what your starting point is.

For example, if you have never run before and you are preparing for your first marathon or half marathon, regardless of how many weeks you have been following the plan, there should be small amounts of intensity a couple of times a week; if there are long runs with tempos, these are not for you. This is something that Damian only introduced to my training a few years ago – and remember that I have been running for twenty years.

It all goes back to having the right framework and strength in place to support this type of running. While your body might manage it once or twice, if you have never run at a faster pace before and suddenly start doing a lot, the cracks – quite literally – will start to show in your body.

CASE STUDY

A twenty-four-year-old female training for the London Marathon came to work with me after she had picked up an injury. It wasn't anything too serious, but it was enough to stop her running for a few weeks, and she was informed enough to know that things could be worse the next time if she didn't seek some professional support. She also admitted that her menstrual cycle had changed since starting on the training plan.

She had started running six months previously and had signed up with a well-established running app. The onboarding process involved adding her personal information, age, sex and address, and then what her goal was.

There were no questions about her previous running or even fitness experience. There was nothing asking her about her injury history, menstrual cycle or general lifestyle, apart from if she was a smoker or not.

She was set up with a marathon plan and when she shared it with me, I was quite shocked. It ramped up pretty quickly, especially in intensity. In addition, she was doing all her running before work and before breakfast, so it didn't really surprise me that she had become injured, or that her menstrual cycle had been affected.

We introduced a pre-training snack of either a banana, a glass of juice or, if she was really struggling, half a gel before she ran, with the other half during her run. We also discussed her work and lifestyle, and agreed that she should shorten some of the higher-intensity sessions.

She did make it round the London Marathon and her menstrual cycle returned to normal relatively quickly after my input, but we agreed that moving forward it would be best for her to work with an actual running coach who could tailor her training to her goals and her lifestyle in order to support both health and performance.

Sadly, this was not an isolated incident with this particular running app. During the first half of 2024, I worked with twelve people who had suffered some form of injury, ranging from repeated niggles as in the case study above to severe debilitating stress fractures, or presented with a decline in their metabolic and hormonal health. I spoke to several physios about the training plans and they all showed huge concern. We all individually reached out to the running app with our concerns, but at the time of writing, while our concerns have been registered, there has been no sign of improvements or changes to their onboarding information or practice.

CHAPTER 3

Let's talk about sports nutrition

Nutrition is not complex, but it is a topic of great controversy.

In my last book, *More Fuel You* (see contents pages), I discussed a number of controversial nutrition topics and provided up-to-date scientific information to help you find the right nutritional approach based on your needs.

While I aim to explain many of the common themes associated with food, eating and running in this chapter, I don't just want to repeat what I have previously written in *More Fuel You*, especially around sports nutrition theory. There will of course also be some overlap, as science hasn't changed significantly in the last few years. For those of you who have already read *More Fuel You*, the following chapters continue the discussion almost like a part 2. For those of you who haven't read it (why not? Joke!), you will still be able to follow my words but you may find that you want to read *More Fuel You* for completion.

When it comes to nutrition specifically for performance, it feels like everyone has an opinion, but often this is based solely on their own experience; or the science, when it is available, is simplified to fuelling and recovery.

In reality, human bodies are not machines; while we definitely need fuel to survive, it is not as simple as 'we can cover a certain number of miles when we fill our tank with a specific number of litres of petrol', as with cars. In fact, when you stop and consider human biology, the body is a series of intricate processes that interact and work in conjunction with each other to keep us alive. This is why fuelling is never as simple as just 'energy in versus energy out'. It is about the composition of your diet, the timing of your nutrients and the quantities it takes not just to meet the demands of your training load, but also to continue to drive cellular adaptation and essential biological processes.

While there are always trends and beliefs regarding what makes you a better runner, the key scientific findings demonstrate that it is actually consistency in your training that will improve your outcome.[4]

Although following a diet trend, taking a supplement or fixating on your weight may feel like the path towards optimal performance, many of these are not sustainable or based on any credible evidence, and often result in a break in your training. Ensuring that you make appropriate choices around your training and lifestyle will help you to maintain your training effort day after day, resulting in progression while also helping to maintain motivation and encourage adaptation from your training. Studies have also shown that the timing of nutrition has an integral role to play in hormonal balance, bone health and maintaining your immune system.

IMMUNITY

Staying well is of huge importance for consistent training. However, balancing immunity with higher training loads, full-time work and family life can make this very challenging. Some tips for staying on top of your immunity include:

1 Staying hydrated – saliva is the first line of defence, using electrolytes during the summer months and also during the winter months if you are doing any training indoors on the treadmill or in the gym.
2 Maintaining vitamin D levels above 75 nanomoles per litre – which may mean taking vitamin D supplement especially through the winter months (September to April in the northern hemisphere). The maintenance dose I recommend to most of the athletes I work with is 2,000 IU (international units) per day, but I adjust this according to their levels, which I test at least twice a year.
3 Ensuring appropriate iron levels, including ferritin stores of above 50 micrograms per litre, ideally through dietary choices (see chapter 4) but sometimes a supplement will be necessary.

4 Starting a course of probiotics twelve weeks out from your A race – studies have shown that this helps to reduce the risk of upper respiratory tract infections in athletes.[5]

5 Sleep – aim for a minimum of eight hours a night to support your immunity. While there is a temptation to reduce sleep in order to fit in extra training, this approach does not pay off in the long term and usually ends up disrupting your training.

It is not your fault if you get confused and subsequently find yourself in a place where your fuelling is inadequate and negatively impacts both your health and performance. As repeatedly stated both here and in *More Fuel You*, the world of nutrition is a confusing one, with messages coming from multiple sources. While most of us are becoming increasingly aware that not everything we read on social media is true or credible, how do we navigate those nutritional guidelines that seemingly come from respected resources in the form of public health messaging? From billboards to leaflets in our doctor's surgery to television adverts, what and how we eat is big news.

Do we all need to worry about obesity?

There is no doubt that obesity is on the government's agenda. According to the World Health Organization, in 2022, 43% of adults aged eighteen and over were overweight, and 16% were living with obesity, where obesity is defined as an individual having a BMI of 30 or above.[6] These statistics influence public health messages and societal perceptions.

However, how relevant are these messages if you are among the 84% who are not obese? Even if you fall into the overweight category, your health metrics may not be of concern if you exercise regularly and make mindful food choices. Not everyone categorised as overweight should be labelled as 'unhealthy', as health encompasses more than just weight. Unfortunately, this message often induces fear and shame, leading to unhealthy behaviours.

BMI is the ratio between height and weight, and while it serves as a measure, it is not always the most accurate, with many athletes with a larger but lean frame falling into the overweight category by default, with no consideration given to body composition. However, it is presently the criterion used for weight classification due to the fact that it is easy to collect and non-invasive.

Regardless of the accuracy of using BMI as a marker, we know that being overweight and/or obese carries more risk of developing chronic health conditions. Thus, the key focus of public health nutrition messaging is on this target audience to encourage behaviour change and improve their health metrics.

How do I know if nutrition messages are relevant to me?

While there is sufficient evidence to suggest that we all need to be more mindful of the food we choose – reducing intakes of saturated fat, sugar and salt, and increasing wholegrains, fruits and vegetables – how do we get the balance right when we are also physically very active and have high energy requirements?

Just this morning, I saw a headline pop up on my news feed from a very popular national men's fitness magazine, claiming that a new study had stated that you need to include more fibre and protein in order to sustain weight loss. However, what the article did not go on to explain was that the subject group for this study was people who were sedentary and overweight, not those who were physically active even if they were overweight. Obviously, the media wants to create clickbait articles and often sensationalises headlines, but they also omit key pieces of information, which is misleading and results in changes to behaviours that are not appropriate for the demographic reading the articles.

When you exercise, you stimulate your appetite – a physiological process. Many people resist this urge in order to maintain a calorie deficit for weight loss, but this often leads to failure, with many feeling like they are eating out of control at the end of the day. This evokes feelings of shame and a desperation to overcompensate the next day, setting up a cycle of repeated failure. And yet this is just the body's way of trying to achieve energy balance.

If we look at the messaging around sugar as a specific example, the Scientific Advisory Committee on Nutrition recommends that added sugar should account for no more than 5% of our total daily energy intake, which is the equivalent of 30 grams for adults. In comparison, when we look at endurance running, the recommendation is that for runs above sixty minutes at high intensity or ninety minutes at moderate intensity, we should be consuming 30–60 grams of carbohydrate, ideally glucose and/or fructose to support training by delivering energy to our working muscles (more on this in chapter 4).

Thus, someone who is out doing a two-hour moderate-intensity run would need to take on up to 120 grams of carbohydrate to help maintain their pace, spare glycogen stores and try to counteract that cardiovascular stress we discussed in chapter 2. This is before taking into consideration their recovery needs. All of this makes following government guidance difficult if you want to actually support your training and performance.

In fact, this is one of the most common mistakes I witness in my clinic: individuals who are trying to adhere to what they deem healthy eating, while also training hard with a specific performance goal in mind. In a lot of cases, following healthy-eating guidance leads to under-fuelling, poor performance and, in extreme cases, difficult and dysfunctional relationships with food.

Popularity and notoriety

Those of you who know me well and follow my educational messaging on social media will know that I have a tendency to call out misinformation and poor practice. While writing this book I had recently seen many individuals in my clinic who had signed up for bespoke nutrition apps but had been given advice that had left them metabolically in a real pickle.

There is a long list of companies and brands which claim to provide individualised and bespoke dietary approaches to improve health. They offer continuous glucose monitoring and gut microbiome testing and other such tech. They have gained a lot of momentum and trust. So what is the problem, I hear you ask?

Despite their bold claims and affiliations, there are big flaws and issues with the scientific data these apps present to back up their practices. In particular, they fail to take into consideration all the factors that impact blood glucose and overlook the fact that food is not the only thing that causes our glucose levels to fluctuate or even spike. In fact, we know that stress (think fight or flight), illness, the menstrual cycle, dehydration and physical activity all contribute to this. Indeed, a number of case studies have shown that even when individuals eat exactly the same food daily for a week, their blood glucose fluctuates significantly.[7] This demonstrates that blood glucose is not just as simple as what we eat.

GLUCOSE MONITORING

Until recently, the use of continuous glucose monitors (CGMs) was only used and discussed in clinical settings, generally within the type 1 diabetic population. Type 1 diabetics have a lifelong condition where their pancreas doesn't produce insulin as a result of an autoimmune condition. This is usually detectable at a young age, and these individuals need to be given insulin extrinsically. In this situation, monitoring glucose is advantageous to support appropriate administration of insulin throughout the day.

The human body is a series of chemical reactions that work on feedback loops. In individuals without type 1 diabetes, the body has the ability to regulate blood glucose within normal limits using the hormones glucagon and insulin.

When we consume carbohydrates, we break these down into glucose and this is then stored in our muscles, liver and brain in the form of glycogen until the body needs it as an energy source. When glucose levels drop, glucagon releases glucose; and when glucose levels rise, insulin is released by the pancreas and this lowers glucose levels by directing the glucose into storage within the body. This monitoring process is part of homeostasis that occurs in the body. Ironically, it is the body's own continuous glucose monitoring.

While the human body likes to keep blood glucose levels within a certain range, this is not an absolute number and this becomes an issue when using a CGM. It starts to create fear and anxiety. Due to scaremongering, you start to believe that something terrible will happen if your blood glucose is one point off what is deemed 'normal'. However, clinical data shows that it is actually normal for blood glucose levels to fluctuate a lot throughout the day. In fact, in healthy individuals without type 1 diabetes, it is normal for blood glucose levels to sit out of normal range (4 to 7.8 millimoles per litre) for short periods of time without any adverse consequences to health.

This may become a problem if an individual's blood glucose remains chronically elevated as a result of insulin resistance. However, contrary to all the media messaging, this is not something that affects everyone. It is associated with type 2 diabetes, which can occur as a result of some genetic predisposition, a sedentary lifestyle and individuals holding more adipose (body fat) around their trunk region. It is a condition that can be reversed by improved lifestyle behaviours, and these individuals are potentially the only group of people who may benefit from some of these apps.

Similarly, to date, we don't actually know what the 'ideal' gut microbiome looks like. Dr Rob Knight, one of the leading voices in the field of gut health, states: 'There's a lot of healthy microbiomes and they have almost nothing in common.'

Thus, there really is no way of testing and comparing an individual's gut microbiome against a gold standard. Additionally, the gut microbiome varies so much depending on cultural background, hormonal status, lifestyle factors and antibiotic use that we can't even say that testing someone's stool is an accurate reflection of their overall gut health, as it just gives us a snapshot for that specific moment in time. Finally, the science is not robust enough at this stage to claim that we need to eat in a certain way to increase levels of certain bacteria to reduce our risk of a certain condition or disease, as claimed by some apps.

There are definitely benefits to eating more wholegrains and fibre in general, but as I discuss in chapter 4, this is not always relevant to those of us who run.

GLUCOSE AND RUNNING

When we run, blood glucose typically rises from 5 millimoles to 10 millimoles to ensure that glucose can be transported to the working muscles. However, if you were monitoring this using a CGM, you would also see that blood glucose would drop within a few minutes as a direct action of exercise. In fact, this is why type 1 diabetics have to be mindful when administering their insulin and timing their nutrition when exercising. They have to try to mimic the intricate process and control that occurs naturally within the body.

CASE STUDY

Earlier this year, I worked with a forty-three-year-old female runner with type 1 diabetes who wanted some advice ahead of a multi-day trail race. She presented with a complex medical history and understandably had some real anxieties about her blood glucose values. These had been further impacted by scaremongering and media messaging around glucose spikes. She had recently moved over to using a CGM, which had further elevated her anxieties as she could see the numbers all the time. However, she had not been aware of the impact of training and other factors such as dehydration, stress and hormonal health that also played into these values. Incidentally, she had been restricting her intake of carbohydrate, feeling terrible but also being surprised that her blood glucose was still often high.

What she had not appreciated was that when we don't fuel our bodies appropriately, this increases our production of stress hormones. These actually cause more glucose to be released into the body, thus registering high levels.

We spent a couple of sessions playing around with her nutritional intake to support her training, but I also encouraged her to hold her nerve when it came to her insulin administration, especially when she saw elevated levels immediately after a training session. There is a lag period associated with the body catching up, where the impact of training also has a blood glucose lowering effect.

She emailed me recently to tell me that the advice had paid off and she had exceeded her expectations in the race, even managing a podium finish.

Remember that glucose is the preferred currency of the body and especially the brain. And while it's best to consume complex carbs that can be broken down into glucose, in certain situations like during and after endurance and high-intensity exercise, easily digestible options are preferable to support performance and recovery. Here, taking on simple carbohydrates results in a blood glucose spike, which releases insulin, and this process allows glucose to be drawn back into the muscles and replenish glycogen stores.

Regardless of the lack of credible and appropriate science or data to back their claims, my biggest problem with some of these apps is their lack of transparency about who their product is actually suitable for. They might claim that their product is not suitable for anyone who is physically active or anyone with a history of a dysfunctional relationship with food, but all the individuals I had seen in my clinic had been open about their involvement with sport or even a specific goal such as marathon training before signing up to the apps.

How can we achieve balance?

There are always going to be nutrition and fitness trends which we have to learn to navigate. Likewise, public health messaging is here to stay. While this does not in any way mean you should discard all public health nutritional guidance, it does encourage you to consider what is appropriate and relevant to your circumstances.

If you have taken up running as a way of keeping fit and improving weight and other health metrics, such as high blood pressure, then being mindful about your sugar, salt and saturated fat intake are still going to be important considerations. However, if you are an established runner with no concern about health metrics, while this doesn't give you the green light to eat sugar for breakfast, lunch and dinner, or even suggest that it's fine to consume highly processed foods, it does show that you have to find a nutritional approach that fits with your needs, lifestyle and training. I discuss this and lots more in *More Fuel You*.

Can we lose weight while we are exercising?

Many people start running as a way of trying to control or lose weight. Exercise and weight loss is an interesting topic. There have been numerous studies indicating that exercise alone is not sufficient to result in weight loss. One simple reason is that when we move more, it stimulates our appetite. As humans, we are biologically biased to want to achieve energy balance, so we tend to respond to this increase in appetite. Similarly, it has been shown that if we see exercise as a means to lose weight, it often becomes a chore or even a punishment. Instead, if we see exercise for its health and well-being benefits, we are more likely to be successful at sticking to it, and this has many more benefits in the long term, such as improved blood pressure, cardiovascular health, bone health and also mood.[8, 9]

One of the questions I am asked the most frequently is whether it is possible to lose weight while also training for a performance outcome at a specific event. My first question back is usually, 'why do you want to lose weight?' Nine times out of ten, the response is because 'lighter makes you faster!' I usually finish off the sentence: ' … until it doesn't.'

Weight loss is a complex subject, both physiologically and psychologically. There is no doubt that in the Western world there is a societal bias towards a particular body type, a body size. The general narrative that is loud and present, despite campaigns to change attitudes, is that a smaller body is more acceptable. And yet our body size tells us very little about the person we are. As I often say, 'Your body is the least interesting thing about you!'

Does fitness/athleticism have a look?

Historically, we associate running with a particular body type. While many athletes defy this norm, especially away from road running, they are often less celebrated.

The images we are bombarded with inform our thoughts and beliefs, but it is important to appreciate that elite-level athletes tend to be genetic outliers – their bodies are naturally that way. In order to achieve fast times again and again, they have to fuel correctly, train appropriately and rest sufficiently.

Have you ever stopped to think about those athletes who post one great performance and then are never seen or heard of again? Or those athletes who stay on the scene but are plagued with injury after injury? These athletes may be genetically gifted, but they don't fuel sufficiently to be sustainable in their sport.

Is it ever acceptable to lose weight for running performance?

If you legitimately have excess body fat, losing this can indeed improve your running performance, within reason, but there is a lot to consider.

Firstly, you have to understand your body type. Not everyone who runs is going to be long-limbed with naturally low body fat, as often seen in the elite arena, particularly in endurance running. While this body type may be advantageous for running, it doesn't mean it is the only body type that can run.

So many of the runners I work with are already at the optimal set point for their body, but the belief that losing weight or achieving a certain body ideal will make them a better runner can lead to dysfunctional behaviours.

The human body is a series of chemical reactions. Each of these needs energy to be maintained and an optimal environment to work efficiently. Collectively, these chemical reactions create a metabolic environment.

When we over-restrict our nutritional intake, or create too big a deficit by also training hard, there may be initial changes to our body mass. However, if this is rapid, the majority of loss is muscle mass, not body fat. Muscle mass actually weighs more than body fat, but it takes up less space, generates more power and speed and is also metabolically active, and so this is the component of body composition that we really want to preserve.

Similarly, when we create too big a deficit or try to drop our weight too far below our natural set point, the body goes into compensatory behaviours and down-regulates metabolism in order to preserve energy. Thus, contrary to what we often read, reducing energy intake doesn't always result in weight loss and can actually cause an individual to hold on to more body fat.

It is also important to remember that exercise such as running stimulates appetite and has a metabolic response associated with it. After we exercise, if we fuel appropriately and provide our body with sufficient energy intake, the body will use this to increase metabolic activity while it repairs, restores and responds to the stimulus that is training. If we don't provide our body with enough energy for the training we are demanding of it, it can't engage in these metabolic processes, so the individual can't repair and restore appropriately, increasing their risk of injury and poor performance and also preventing them from losing weight.

So in reality, if you are running to lose weight, especially if you are new to running, just the very act of running without changing your diet is likely to lead to changes in your body mass and composition. As time goes on, you will need to adjust your nutritional intake, especially as you put down more lean muscle mass, in order to fuel your running appropriately and keep seeing the benefits to your body composition until they reach a place that is optimal for you.

When I'm working with runners, especially those who want to lose weight, I start by asking what their most desired outcome is. Do they value weight loss more than overall performance? Nine out of ten clients choose performance as their preferred outcome. Indeed, when they trust the process and allow me to advise on how to eat for performance – that is, fuelling appropriately around their training to ensure those cellular adaptations – their body composition improves as a result, and they usually stand on the start line at the right body composition for them for optimal performance.

This is definitely the approach I take. Damian, Germain and Elsey are the same. They may well have periods of time when they are not working towards an A race where they are a little more relaxed with their nutritional approach. However, once they are in full training mode and working towards a specific goal, they pay more attention and ensure that they adapt their nutritional intake to their training volume and intensity, and their body composition adapts accordingly.

So what and how should you eat?

The key is to ensure that you fuel up with good sources of complex carbs ahead of your training runs, especially those that are longer or higher intensity. I'm not just talking about the meal immediately ahead of the session, but about your nutritional intake twenty-four to thirty-six hours ahead. Additionally, it is important to recover immediately afterwards with both carbohydrate and protein. Ideally, this would be your next meal, but if it is going to be over an hour until you can consume this meal and you have another training session within twelve hours, this may need to be a recovery drink or snack followed by a meal. If, however, your next training session is twenty-four hours or more later, then recovery can be your next meal.

Timing and composition of diet make a huge difference and reap more rewards than avoiding fuelling altogether. We will go into the theory and practical application of this in part 2. While many people are confused by this, it demonstrates that when we are physically active, the societal messaging of 'move more and eat less' actually needs to be replaced by 'move more and eat more', even when improved body composition is the key goal. Contrary to what we read and hear in mainstream media, this has been the finding of numerous physiological studies on humans and energy balance. But the multi-million-pound diet industry doesn't benefit from our successes, only our failures.

Indeed, the biggest mistake I see in the running world is when individuals focus on weight over performance. By fixating on weight, you influence your behaviour, especially around fuel, and often end up under-fuelling and putting your body and central nervous system under stress, which in turn causes your body to work against you, not for you.

Those who get hung up on a particular ideal and associate this with improved performance often find themselves adopting dysfunctional behaviours. While this is not always conscious, it is driven by a belief and often results in them holding their body at a place that is suboptimal, where it can't work appropriately for them. Over time, their performance also suffers, first stagnating and eventually deteriorating.

CASE STUDY

Several years ago, I worked with a young fell runner. She was a smart young woman who knew the importance of fuelling and having a menstrual cycle for her performance. She had come from a background of consistent injuries as a junior runner, due to overtraining and overcompeting.

She was now working with a really responsible coach who had suggested she come and talk to me. While her performance was improving and she was getting some great outcomes, including podiums at a lot of races, she was really struggling with her body image. She told me that while she rationally knew that being lighter was not the answer for her, she found it really difficult at the start of races because she felt a lot larger than the others around her, and this was niggling away at her. What if she could drop some weight – would it give her that edge?

We talked about her general experience and she appreciated that every time she tried to restrict her energy intake, her performance faltered rather than improved and she usually ended up getting injured. I asked her to consider this evidence.

While it took a few sessions, over time she started to see that while her body did not fit her idea of what a good runner looked like, in reality her performances suggested that she was actually at the optimal place for her based on her genetics and she was getting great results.

Beliefs, societal pressures and ideals

Food is so much more than fuel.

Daily in my clinic, I hear from those who struggle with a difficult and complex relationship with food. They are constantly weighing up whether they should or shouldn't eat something, worrying about potential consequences that in reality will not happen and yet their anxious mind allows them to believe the worst-case scenario. They feel the need to earn food and don't appreciate just how much energy our bodies need just to stay alive before we even take a step out of bed in the morning.

It fills me with sadness that so many of us live by rules and external cues of what we should eat, rather than what our bodies, hearts and minds tell us we want and often need. Modern society has a lot to answer for. I am reminded of this every time I go back to one of my favourite countries, Nepal. It is a country where survival, being grateful for a roof over your head and running water are the main focus, and worrying about 'being successful' or 'adopting a lifestyle in order to be accepted' are far from the list of priorities. Yet in Western society, many of us feel a general unease and discomfort, a sense of unworthiness and inadequacy of never quite meeting the mark. The constant stream of images through social media; the influential voices of those we put on a pedestal playing into our subconscious, suggesting that we are not quite enough. We must do more, we must be more and we must work towards an ideal in order to feel good about ourselves. We go in pursuit of body compositions, job successes, academic and sporting achievements, trying to attain what we can't find within ourselves – that is, self-worth. But who is to say that these ideals we constantly compare ourselves to are right for us? How do we know?

One of the key features of beauty is being able to embrace being unique and not constantly feeling that you have to merge into what everyone else perceives as acceptable. The most attractive individuals are the ones who are truly comfortable in their own skin, the ones who unconditionally accept themselves, flaws and all.

Many of us create limiting beliefs that provide us with this false refuge that 'we are safe', but in reality, can restricting or avoiding food, pushing the body to extremes and constantly cracking the whip really be something we can define as 'safe'?

From my years of experience, both professional and personal, I think the biggest challenge we face as humans is dealing with uncertainty – the fear of the unknown and wanting control over situations and outcomes we have absolutely no control over. We can't control someone's response to a situation, no matter how much we restrict our food intake. We can't change the outcome of a given situation, no matter how much we train, so why do we believe that we have a sense of control?

In reality, we are only in control when we have choice – when we can choose what we really want to eat for breakfast, lunch and dinner; when we choose what type of movement we want to do today based on how our body is feeling. In fact, wanting control over every aspect of our life sets us up to fail, as we create unrealistic expectations and standards that will never be met.

My story

While this is my story, it could be that of so many that I work with – not the exact experiences I went through but the underlying nature of why someone ends up with a dysfunctional relationship with food and their body.

I developed anorexia when I was thirteen years old. It wasn't a conscious decision as such, but over the years I have understood why it developed and what those behaviours gave me. All I remember is feeling a deep-rooted unease within my body. Now I appreciate that this was associated with a feeling of not belonging, a sense of falling short, being a constant disappointment and a deep sense of self-loathing. Fundamentally, I did not fit. As a teenager, it was far easier for me to blame everything on my body. That is what so many of us do: project our insecurities on to our body because this is actually something we can try to mould, control and even contain.

I can also see now that anorexia was my way of making my body as small and insignificant as the world around me made me feel. It was an opportunity to express my anger – I felt lost, abandoned and misunderstood, so it was my way of sticking two fingers up to those around me and in my own way saying, 'I don't need anything from any of you. I don't even need food!' Again, none of this was conscious or made sense at the time. I just walked around believing that I would be more acceptable and lovable if my body fitted. My weight plummeted, and so did my personality. I withdrew from the world, isolated myself. My world became: get up, go to school, survive school, get home and avoid eating dinner, go to bed and repeat. It was a miserable existence and not one I would wish on anyone.

While I physically restored weight and 'recovered' relatively quickly, I was far from okay. During my time recovering at the Maudsley Hospital, I learnt nothing about why I had developed this dysfunctional relationship with food and my body. I just knew that all eyes were on me, and while I didn't feel comfortable in my restored body, I also didn't want to go back to the depths of being so underweight that all you experience is darkness and despair, an isolation and loneliness that no words can do justice to. But I still didn't trust my body or really know how to look after it.

I would say that I was 'functional' for many years, which meant I was showing up at being part of life but my relationship with food was still unhealthy, and my dissatisfaction with my body was high.

But I was also motivated to be well. By this stage, I knew I wanted to be a dietitian and I was aware that I couldn't be one if it was clear that I still had a disordered relationship with food. In those days, to be accepted on the course, you had to attend an interview which involved assessing your relationship with food. Personally, I wish this still stood because I see a shocking number of newly qualified dietitians and nutritionists who clearly have a very complex relationship with food – but, guess what, they are popular on social media!

I've spoken about this before, but it was my work as a dietitian that really helped me to see food differently. Working with patients who were too sick to be able to swallow or absorb food helped me to realise how privileged I was to be in a position where food was so easily available and accessible to me.

However, it was having my first daughter that really solidified my trust in my body. Watching my body grow and then giving birth, feeding a baby and returning to where my body had been prior to falling pregnant without having to control my diet helped me to appreciate that my body definitely had a set point that worked for me. I'll be honest, my body weight has pretty much stayed exactly the same throughout my adult years, only really changing in body composition depending on how much training I am doing.

That said, when I started running a little more seriously, especially during my road marathon era and probably the first couple of ultras I did, I noticed that my relationship with food and my body altered a little again. This was never to the extreme of my teenage years, but I found myself falling into the same trap as many of my clients around feeling the need to earn my food. The more competitive I became, the more I would feel real anxiety if I didn't run. Gone were the carefree days of running three times a week; now I was out running five times a week minimum, while also looking after two small daughters.

I was frustrated because I noticed that all-too-familiar unease within my body. However, now I was a mum and I wanted to be a good role model. I walked around never feeling very confident or comfortable in my body, but I had learnt not to respond. I can see now, especially when I consider how much I eat today in comparison to those marathon days, that I was under-fuelling, and I'm pretty sure this also contributed to the stress on my body that led to that sarcoidosis and burnout diagnosis.

But here is the thing I discuss with my clients now: when life feels chaotic and messy, for whatever reason, we always go back to the place we have been to before in order to 'feel okay'. And while this gives us a temporary reprieve, it is never the answer and often just leads to more problems, usually negative consequences for our physical health. So many of us chase these false refuges in the hope that they will be the solution to why we don't feel okay or why we don't fit, but in reality they just take us further and further away from the person we truly are.

So what changed for me? How did I get to a place where food, body and exercise no longer was or is troublesome? Many factors have contributed to this. Becoming more self-aware and gaining a real understanding of my personality. Appreciating that I do have quite a dominant critical self, and while this side of me tends to call out all my flaws, this is just based on beliefs and the old story that I grew up with. I know that I have a choice in how I respond, and mostly I choose not to believe the false content my mind is dictating. Similarly, I have become aware of scenarios and situations that make me more vulnerable, and while I don't avoid these, I know that I need to be a bit more vigilant about my thoughts, feelings and then potential behaviours.

Knowledge has also had a huge part to play. This comes from my work, the additional training and qualifications to understand human behaviour, working in the field of REDs (see chapter 8) and contributing to academic publications, but also my personal experience of appreciating that when I fuel to train, I actually feel stronger, train better and notice the adaptation and progression.[10, 11]

I got to a place over twenty years ago when I started to trust my body, and I live by this. I listen and respond. I know that the human body knows what to do and has its own inbuilt monitoring tool. Ever since I tuned into this, I have been in balance and liberated from a need to control. I know where my body needs to be physically in order to perform well, and while that may not conform with body ideals associated with fitness, it is absolutely the right place for my body to perform optimally.

Final word

Before we move into part 2 and discuss the specifics of fuelling and how to bring it all to life practically, I want to remind you all that there are three fundamental factors regardless of your running goal:
1. Even if you are pursuing a time or distance goal, don't forget to focus on running for enjoyment and the social connections.
2. Learn to trust your body and listen to it. Fuel appropriately and watch how, over time, it improves not just in performance but also in body composition.
3. Be mindful of the noise and focus on advice that is relevant to you and your personal circumstances.

PART 2

Putting it into practice

CHAPTER 4

The store cupboard

What do runners need? As we have discussed briefly, the amount, composition and timing of nutrition is important to support a runner with their performance outcomes. While runners should base their diet around key healthy-eating guidelines, the volumes and amounts will vary widely and will depend on training volume and intensity. Additionally, there are certain key nutrients that play an important role in performance but are often overlooked.

Carbohydrates

Carbohydrate is the key fuel source for exercise as it is broken down into glucose, the body's preferred currency, and utilised by the body to provide energy.

Carbohydrate is stored as glycogen throughout the body, but specifically within the liver and muscles. It is this source within the muscles that is the most readily available energy for working muscles, releasing energy more quickly than other sources. However, this storage facility is limited. If the muscles are inadequately fuelled, this will lead to fatigue and poor performance, placing additional stress on the nervous system and immune health, and potentially putting us at greater risk of injury and illness.

To give you some context, it takes around 500 grams of carbohydrate in males and 400 grams in females to have completely full muscle glycogen stores, with an additional 80 grams in liver glycogen, mainly used to maintain energy to the brain. When muscle glycogen is at full capacity, at most this will last around 90–120 minutes when running at around 65–75% of your maximal heart rate. The quicker you go, the faster your stores will deplete. Thus, if you train most days, your glycogen stores will always be slightly depleted.

This helps to explain how important it is to plan your carbohydrate intake around and during training sessions: the amount you require will be dependent on the frequency, duration and intensity of your training. However, regardless of what you may have read, exercise and running uses a lot of energy.

The present sport nutrition recommendations associated with carbohydrate are as follows:

- For low-intensity or rest days, requirements are around 3 grams of carbohydrate per kilogram of body weight per day.
- For an hour of moderate training a day, requirements are around 5–7 grams per kilogram of body weight per day.
- For training one to three hours a day, requirements are 6–10 grams per kilogram of body weight per day.
- For training four to six hours a day over multiple sessions, requirements are 8–12 grams per kilogram of body weight per day.

As a caveat for anyone who is training a minimum of four times a week and/or including some double days to include resistance training or other cross-training such as climbing, you may need to keep your carbohydrate intake higher than 3 grams per kilogram of body weight even on rest days to ensure that you recover appropriately but also start refuelling for your next run day (more on this in chapter 6).

To help you meet your needs, it is important to understand the difference in the available types of carbohydrate. Over the years, carbohydrates have been classified in many ways, and the most common types are simple and complex.

Simple carbohydrates include dairy, fruit and sugar, honey and molasses. Complex carbohydrates are those including pasta, rice, oats, couscous, potatoes, bread and cereals. Runners need a mix of both – ideally complex carbohydrates at mealtimes and then more simple options immediately before, during and after training, depending on the training session.

We will look at the practical application of this around specific training in chapter 6.

Fruit and vegetables

We are all being encouraged to eat more fruit and vegetables for our overall health and also for our digestive health. However, one of the most common mistakes I see is individuals assuming that vegetables count as carbohydrate and thus provide our bodies with energy.

To explain this better, we need to talk about calories and how not all calories are equal. Humans, and runners in particular, also need to move on from the misconceptions around 'calories in' versus 'calories out'.

A calorie is defined as the amount of heat needed to raise the temperature of 1 gram of water by 1 degree Celsius. Thus, a calorie is a unit of energy or heat that arises from the combustion of the nutritional components of our diet.

We need calories to provide us with the energy required to live; every single biological process in the body requires energy and this has to come from the food we eat, which gets broken down to yield energy. So we also need energy in the form of calories to support our running endeavours.

The problem is that humans are not calorimeters and how we utilise food is very different from calories just being burnt and providing energy. If we take the humble carrot, calorie tables tell us that 100 grams of carrots provide us with 10 calories. While this is true when you burn carrots in a calorimeter, it is not the same in a human. Carrots are predominantly indigestible by the human gut, so when we consume 100 grams of carrots, we only actually absorb a very small amount of those 10 calories. This is problematic for those of us who are physically active, as if we consume too many vegetables, we may displace our intake of carbohydrate and struggle to consume the actual amount of energy we need to support our body.

CASE STUDY

I recently worked with a young woman who had only really been running for a year. Prior to that, she described herself as someone who was overweight, sedentary and didn't really care about what she was eating. Influenced by social media, she started to make some changes to her diet and took up running at the same time. Initially, the changes to her body composition were slow, but she started to feel more confident in herself. Buoyed on by more and more compliments, she continued to use Instagram as her source of information, which resulted in her replacing carbs with fruit and vegetables. So, for example, her evening meals would consist of a piece of chicken and a load of vegetables, even though she had run 10 kilometres beforehand. What she had not appreciated is how important carbohydrates are not just for energy and recovery but also for bone health, specifically bone activity post-exercise.[12]

When she presented to me, she had been diagnosed with a stress fracture of the neck of femur which had occurred three months previously, only nine months after starting running and restricting her intake, specifically her carbohydrate intake. Her consultant had referred her to me to see if we could work together to improve her nutritional intake and support the recovery of her stress fracture.

Thankfully, although she was a little unsure about reintroducing carbohydrates, especially due to all the scaremongering on social media, she had also learnt a lot from her experience and was keen to move forward with healthier and more sustainable behaviours to support her running.

She has since been given the all-clear to start loading her hip, and although she knows she may have to be patient to restart running, she is doing everything she can to ensure that she doesn't encounter similar injuries in the future. She has introduced carbohydrates to all her meals and is also re-educating herself on the amount of fuel she needs to maintain her present weight, which is at a healthy place for her and also supports her running.

Proteins

Proteins are often called the building blocks of the body. They consist of combinations of structures called amino acids. There are twenty amino acids and these combine in various sequences to make muscles, bones, tendons, skin, hair and other tissues. They serve other functions as well, including transporting nutrients and producing enzymes. Eight of these amino acids are essential and must come from our diet. They are found as a complete source in animal-protein food such as dairy, meat, fish and eggs. They are found in an incomplete source in plant-based proteins such as vegetables, grains, nuts and legumes. These are 'incomplete' because they lack one or more of the essential amino acids. However, if they are combined in the correct way, you can make a whole source of protein. Some good combinations include baked beans on toast, rice and dhal, and wholegrain bagels with peanut butter.

We hear a lot about protein within the sports and fitness industry, with many of us believing it to be the most important macronutrient for active individuals. In reality, runners need protein primarily as a response to exercise rather than as a fuel source. The exception to the rule is long ultras of more than 100 kilometres or where the trail involves high levels of downhill running. It has been suggested that regular intakes of protein in these instances can mitigate some muscle damage. The recommendation is 5–10 grams of protein per hour but, as with all sports nutrition, finding the sweet spot for each athlete is key.[13] Remember that protein is harder to digest and absorb than carbohydrate, so how much and what an individual runner can tolerate will vary. When I work with athletes, I tend to start with 20–30 grams of protein every four to six hours and then finalise their race-day strategy based on their feedback (more on this in chapter 6).

Protein has been a huge area of research for many years, with the most recent findings demonstrating how important it is in the recovery phase. I will talk about the specifics and give practical suggestions in chapter 6.

During all exercise – including endurance sports such as running and cycling, and team or power sports such as netball, football, tennis or resistance training (using weights) – an increase in the breakdown of protein in the muscle has been shown. That said, while there is a preference to include a large amount of protein in the immediate recovery phase, the recommendations are that protein foods should be distributed throughout the day, to help counteract a negative protein balance.

The suggested amount is 0.4 grams of protein per kilogram of body weight four to six times a day depending on training load. Those of us who are over forty years old will need to consume higher amounts of protein to support our recovery. There is a whole chapter on masters athletes in *More Fuel You*, but in general I would suggest 0.4 grams of protein per kilogram of body weight every three hours.[14]

Do we need protein supplements?

As we know, protein is a macro that gets a lot of attention. In recent years, it has been given almost an evangelical status; as long as a food contains protein, it is somehow good and healthy for us, even if it is associated with types of food that are deemed non-nutrient-dense, such as ice cream or chocolate bars.

Don't get me wrong, I have nothing against the occasional bowl of ice cream or eating chocolate; in fact, as my close friends know, I rarely deny myself chocolate (Cadbury's Wispa bites, Tony's milk creamy hazelnut crunch or Ritter's dark chocolate and hazelnut, for those asking!). However, I do have to draw the line and say that even with protein added, these products don't suddenly become nutrient-dense choices.

So how can we ensure that we meet our requirements?

Aim to include a protein source at every meal. This could be meat, fish, eggs, tofu, nuts, beans or dairy. Personally, I find the texture and taste of many protein powders quite synthetic and I tend to use cow's milk products for recovery. However, professionally, in certain situations it can be beneficial to start to include either a whey protein or plant-based alternative, especially when combined with cow's milk (or oat if you are plant-based) as a good recovery drink post-training. It's particularly useful when it isn't possible to sit down to a proper balanced meal or snack within thirty minutes of finishing your run. However, protein shakes and powders are not cheap, and for those of us watching the pennies, my top tip is to use skimmed milk powder. You can fortify a pint of milk by adding a 55-gram serving of skimmed milk powder to it, which adds a further 20 grams of protein. Like protein powder, you can add skimmed milk powder to porridge and smoothies, but it also has the versatility to be mixed in with savoury sauces and mashed potato.

Where I do think we have to be mindful is with protein bars. They are not all bad – in fact, options like TREK protein flapjacks, Eat Natural and Nature Valley protein bars can be found in my store cupboard. However, I would suggest ditching any protein bars that are full of unrecognisable ingredients and are usually carbohydrate-free. Instead, here are some other options for higher-protein snacks:

- Greek yoghurt with berries and honey
- smoked mackerel pâté on oatcakes
- hummus with carrot and cheese sticks
- toasted crumpet topped with peanut butter and a glass of cow's milk or soya milk
- banana and quark topped with crumbled digestive or ginger biscuits
- seeded oatcakes.

Fat

Contrary to popular belief, not all fat is bad for you. In fact, it is vital that everyone eats some fat to help absorb fat-soluble vitamins A, D, E and K and to provide essential fatty acids that the body cannot make. These nutrients have important roles to play within the body, particularly with regard to recovery, immune health, inflammation and prevention of fatigue.

However, like protein, fat is best reserved for inclusion as an integral part of your daily diet and it should be avoided as an immediate fuel source. In fact, it is worth being aware that a high-fat option pre-run slows digestion and can actually sit heavily on the stomach.

Eating too much of a particular kind of fat – saturated fat – can raise your cholesterol, which increases the risk of heart disease. Saturated fat is the kind of fat found in butter and lard, pies, cakes and biscuits/cookies, fatty cuts of meat, sausages and bacon, cheese and cream. It also encompasses trans fat, which is often found in processed foods. It is important to cut down on this type of fat and choose foods that contain unsaturated fat in preference. These include:

- oily fish, such as salmon, sardines and mackerel, which are an exceptionally good source of omega-3 fatty acids
- nuts and seeds, including their oils and butters
- sunflower, rapeseed and olive oils
- avocados.

When I work with runners, I like to encourage them to use these good fats as much as possible in their diets over saturated varieties. However, it is important to point out that these good fats still have a high energy value and should be eaten with that in mind. One exception to the rule is the saturated fat in dairy – specifically milk, cheese and yoghurt – which has actually been shown to have protective properties for the cardiovascular system.

Vitamins and minerals

Micronutrients are essential for many metabolic processes within the body, but you can't make them yourself and you need to get them from your diet. Most function as coenzymes or cofactors within the body – that is, they aid enzymes and proteins in their function. For example, the B vitamins are very important for carbohydrate and fat metabolism, while vitamin C, along with zinc, is important for a healthy immune system. Magnesium and calcium are needed for muscle contraction.

Do runners have higher requirements of minerals and vitamins? Do they warrant supplementation? The jury is out on this one. Some studies show that there are enhanced requirements in runners due to an increase in damage to muscles by components known as free radicals. However, there have been no absolute links to actual improved sporting performance with a diet high in antioxidants.

So, back to the question of whether runners have higher requirements. Technically no, as it is assumed that people who are physically active will have higher appetites and thus consume more food. As long as this fuel is balanced, nutrient-rich and not made up purely of non-nutrient-dense foods, then you will meet your increased requirements. The exceptions are vegan and vegetarian runners, who may need to pay special attention to certain nutrients such as iron, B12 and omega-3 fatty acids that are difficult to obtain from a predominantly plant-based diet.

As a side note, remember that all forms of fruit, vegetables, herbs and spices count. Personally, I am a big fan of frozen fruit and vegetables, as well as both fresh and dried herbs. Frozen fruit and vegetables are convenient, versatile and actually retain more nutrient density, as they are often picked and then frozen immediately. When I have been travelling with work, it is always a bonus to know that I have a freezer full of vegetables that I can quickly turn into a nutritious meal, especially when I get home late and there is no time to go to the shops.

Here are a few of my go-to frozen fruit and veg options:

OMELETTE
Oil
Couple of handfuls of frozen veg
2–3 eggs (depending on how hungry I am)
Salt, pepper, chilli flakes (optional)
Pinch of herbes de Provence
Cheese (optional)

- Shallow fry the frozen veg in a pan with the oil.
- Meanwhile, beat the eggs and add your seasoning of choice.
- When the veg is cooked, pour the egg mix over the top.
- Once the bottom of the omelette is solid, top with cheese and place under the grill until the top is also firm and the cheese is golden brown.
- Serve with toast or pitta.

CHUNKY SOUP

Oil
2 handfuls of frozen veg
Tin of chickpeas
Carton of plain soup, such as tomato and basil or carrot and coriander
Sriracha sauce

- Cook the veg and chickpeas together in a pan with the oil.
- Once cooked, add the soup and squeeze in a small amount of sriracha sauce.
- Allow to simmer for a few minutes.
- Serve with chunky bread.

BERRY COMPOTE

Individual or mixed frozen berries
Greek yoghurt and honey (optional)

- Place half a packet of frozen berries into a saucepan with a small amount of water at the bottom of the pan.
- Cook over a low heat until the berries have defrosted and been reduced to a thick compote.
- Serve with Greek yoghurt and honey or use as a base for a bircher muesli or topping for pancakes.

Iron

Iron is an important mineral that helps maintain healthy blood. It is a major component of haemoglobin, a type of protein in red blood cells that carries oxygen from your lungs to all parts of your body. Without sufficient iron, there are not enough red blood cells to transport oxygen, leading to fatigue. Thus runners need good iron levels and stores (ferritin) for optimal performance.

Those involved in endurance sports such as running have a higher risk of developing an iron deficiency. This has been reported to impact 3–11% of male athletes and 15–35% of female athletes.[15] There are a number of reasons why this is the case:

- Runners have higher iron requirements due to the increase in production of erythropoietin, which occurs in the bone marrow and is an advantageous training adaptation, optimising performance. This is also the key reason that many elite runners aim to spend some time at high altitude ahead of big races, as altitude accelerates this process.
- Runners also have higher losses of iron due to high training loads that result in hemolysis, which is the breakdown of red blood cells, sweating

- and potential gastrointestinal bleeding, especially during periods of high-intensity training.
- Female runners also have to take into account monthly menstrual losses. While this varies from female to female, most women lose 20–90 millilitres of blood during their period. Those who have heavy periods can have losses in excess of 160 millilitres. It has been stated that up to 14% of women suffer with heavy menstrual bleeding.
- Runners who restrict their nutritional intake and are in low energy availability not only limit their consumption of iron but also compromise absorption and red blood cell production. Low iron storage – that is, low ferritin stores – leads runners to a higher susceptibility to stress fractures.[16]

What are the potential signs of iron deficiency anaemia?

While aerobic metabolism is directly impacted by low iron levels, it has a multifaceted impact. Iron deficiency is associated with:

- reduced overall capacity for strength
- poor coordination
- reduction in power and speed
- a depressed immune system
- increased fatigue
- low mood
- overall reduced recovery.

How is iron deficiency defined?

The Reference Nutrient Intake for dietary iron in the UK is 14.8 milligrams of iron per day for premenopausal women and 8.7 milligrams per day for men and postmenopausal women, with the Recommended Dietary Allowance in the US set at 18 milligrams per day for premenopausal women and 8 milligrams for men and postmenopausal women. While additional iron intakes are recommended for pregnancy and lactation, to date there are no actual additional recommendations for female athletes. However, studies on female runners repeatedly show a need for an additional 10 milligrams of iron per day due to training losses and adaptation.

Iron deficiency can occur with or without anaemia. The World Health Organization defines iron deficiency without anaemia as being when ferritin levels are below 30 micrograms per litre but haemoglobin levels are normal:

above 120 grams per litre in women and 130 grams per litre in men. It defines iron deficiency with anaemia as being when ferritin levels and haemoglobin levels are low.

In sport, we tend to define iron deficiency without anaemia when ferritin levels are below 50 micrograms per litre and haemoglobin labels are above 130 grams per litre for women and 140 grams per litre for men. We define iron deficiency with anaemia when haemoglobin levels are lower than the recommended values.

How can we prevent iron deficiency?

In order to prevent iron deficiency, runners not only need to appreciate that they have higher requirements but also need to know what the best dietary sources are. The best food source of iron is red meat, but many runners have reduced their consumption for other health reasons. Egg yolk is also a good source, but sometimes absorption can be reduced due to the protein in the egg.

Plant-based sources of iron include pulses and legumes, dark green leafy vegetables, nuts and seeds, and foods fortified with iron such as cereal and bread, except wholemeal. In general, iron from plant-based options is much more difficult to absorb. Additionally, foods containing phytates (wholegrains and cereal) and tannins (tea and coffee) impair your absorption of iron. This can be improved by consuming these options with vitamin C or an animal protein, but plant-based runners may need to pay particular attention to their iron intakes.

A good example of how to maximise your iron intake involves combining a cereal such as Bran Flakes with cow's milk, an animal protein, and a source of vitamin C such as a glass of juice or some frozen berries.

In some cases, iron supplementation may be necessary. When supplementing, it is recommended that repeat blood tests should occur six to eight weeks from starting in order to monitor outcome and control the dose.

While it has been proven that the most pronounced effects on iron status by supplementation occur in runners with low ferritin levels, it is clear from the literature that there are no added performance benefits to taking an iron supplement if iron deficiency or iron insufficiency is not indicated. The exception to this is if runners are training at altitude, where supplementation can be of benefit regardless of ferritin stores.

Vitamin D

Vitamin D is a fat-soluble vitamin and hormone produced in the body from sunlight, and is necessary for a number of important biological functions in the body. One of its key roles is increasing intestinal ability to absorb other nutrients, calcium, magnesium and phosphate, which are all involved in bone metabolism.

Vitamin D is also necessary to support muscular recovery and maintain a healthy immune system. It has an important role to play in appetite regulation, and is associated with improved mood, as it is known to increase levels of serotonin. In contrast, vitamin D deficiency will lead to extreme fatigue, increased and prolonged muscle soreness or achy joints, poor recovery between training sessions and low mood.

How much vitamin D do we need?

While we can get small amounts of vitamin D from our diet by eating oily fish and eggs, it is recommended that those of us living in the northern hemisphere take vitamin D supplements through the winter months from September through to April, when available sunlight is limited. The amount tends to depend on our blood levels of vitamin D. For the general population:

- levels of 50 nanomoles per litre or above are adequate for most people for bone and overall health.
- levels below 30 nanomoles per litre are too low and might weaken your bones and affect your health.
- levels above 150 nanomoles per litre are too high and may contribute to health issues.

For runners and those of us who are generally physically active, studies recommend that ideal levels should be above 90 nanomoles per litre but still less than 150 nanomoles per litre. I generally recommend 2000 IU (international units) of vitamin D3 as a maintenance dose. However, if someone has very low levels, then a higher dose protocol will be necessary. Similarly, if someone has high levels of vitamin D, I will reduce or stop supplementation and adjust as needed.

Vitamin B12

This is a key vitamin for everyone but particularly runners, as it contributes to a well-functioning nervous and immune system, alleviates tiredness and fatigue, and maintains healthy blood cells and muscles. Plant-based runners

are particularly at risk of a vitamin B12 deficiency, as it is not available in their diets. Runners with B12 deficiency may experience:
- numbness
- muscle weakness
- psychological issues
- mind and muscle connection balance problems
- painful twitches in the legs and toes.

Unlike the other water-soluble B vitamins that are directly absorbed into the bloodstream from the gut, B12 is bound to protein in food and must be separated before it can be absorbed. This involves a series of complex chemical reactions. When B12 is finally freed, it then combines with intrinsic factor (IF), a glycoprotein in the stomach which allows for full absorption. If B12 is in supplement form, it is already in its free form and does not require the separation stage.

Thus some individuals become deficient due to a lack of production of IF, which can occur as a result of an autoimmune condition, gastric surgery, genetic predisposition or the prolonged use of certain medications such as metformin.

B12 is often absorbed from food by stomach acid, and older runners may also be at a higher risk of developing a B12 deficiency due to a reduction in the production of stomach acid.

How much B12 do we need?

As adults, we need 2.4 micrograms of vitamin B12 a day. The only exceptions are pregnant women, who need 2.6 micrograms a day, and breastfeeding women, who need 2.8 micrograms a day. Runners don't have any extra requirements.

SOURCES OF VITAMIN B12

The best ways to get B12 are from animal sources: dairy, fish, poultry, meat and eggs.
- 1 egg provides 0.5 micrograms of B12.
- 40 grams of cheese provides 0.5 micrograms.
- 250 millilitres of milk provides 1.3 micrograms.

- 90 grams of chicken provides 0.3 micrograms.
- Nutritional yeast is dense in concentration of B12, with 8.3 micrograms per 30-gram serving, but it is important to appreciate that a serving size will be significantly smaller, closer to 3–5 grams.

As previously mentioned, vegan runners should always consider supplementation and aim to be more mindful about using fortified food sources such as cereals to ensure that they meet their daily requirements.

The gut microbiome

The gut microbiome is a topic within the nutrition world that is getting a lot of attention right now. As I mentioned in chapter 3, many brands and organisations are trying to profit from this specialist area, even though we still don't really have enough research to back up the claims they make.

However, we do know that the gut microbiome has an important role to play in our health and well-being. It has a number of functions, including synthesising some vitamins, short-chain fatty acids and even neurotransmitters, all of which are necessary for our physical and mental health.

The area of research that is most widely accepted and discussed is the impact the microbiome has on immune health. Seventy per cent of our immune system resides in our gut.[17] The key appears to be in having diverse gut flora, which can respond to exposure to changes in diet and withstand foreign substances and particles not recognised or tolerated by the body.

Studies have shown that, in general, athletes and those who take part in regular physical activity have more diverse microbiomes than their non-athletic peers. In addition, the type of sport participated in and subsequent diets seem to have a direct impact on the microbiome and gut health.

Endurance athletes who consume a diet rich in complex carbohydrates that helps to meet their energy requirements have been shown to develop a microbiome that helps to reduce inflammation and oxidative stress, thus potentially improving both health and athletic performance.[18] On the flip side, overtraining, under-fuelling and insufficient recovery have been shown to impact the microbiome negatively, resulting in gut dysfunction, increased inflammation and an overall depressed immune system.

While high-fibre diets are being pushed, it is important to remember that for those of us who are physically active, high-fibre diets can displace essential macronutrients such as carbohydrates which are necessary for optimal health and performance.

In fact, this is probably one of the most common mistakes I see in my work: runners with low energy availability (see chapter 8) piling their plates with high-fibre foods which provide volume and help with satiety but don't deliver the energy the body requires for performing, adapting and recovering from sport.

Ergogenic aids

As we have discussed, *how*, *what* and *when* we eat all impact our adaptation and progression. Understanding the fundamentals of a runner's diet is key to optimal performance and prevention of injury. However, many of us are also looking for that extra edge, that product or nutrition approach that promises a small benefit to our performance.

Let's face it, we don't have to look far, as the sports nutrition world promises a whole range of products to improve performance, enhance recovery and reduce fatigue, to name just a few. Indeed, most of the research in sports nutrition is centred around testing novel ingredients to determine how they can improve our performance. While these ergogenic aids may previously have targeted elite and professional athletes, they are now much more mainstream and accessible, but how do we know if they are effective for all of us, regardless of our training background?

Caffeine

In 2021 the International Society of Sports Nutrition updated their position statement on the use of caffeine and exercise performance.[19] The key findings were as follows (taken directly from the paper):

1. Supplementation with caffeine has been shown to acutely enhance various aspects of exercise performance in many but not all studies. Small to moderate benefits of caffeine use include, but are not limited to: muscular endurance, movement velocity and muscular strength, sprinting, jumping, and throwing performance, as well as a wide range of aerobic and anaerobic sport-specific actions.
2. Aerobic endurance appears to be the form of exercise with the most consistent moderate-to-large benefits from caffeine use, although the magnitude of its effects differs between individuals.

3   Caffeine has consistently been shown to improve exercise performance when consumed in doses of 3–6 milligrams per kilogram of body mass. Minimal effective doses of caffeine currently remain unclear but they may be as low as 2 milligrams per kilogram of body mass. Very high doses of caffeine (e.g. 9 milligrams per kilogram) are associated with a high incidence of side-effects and do not seem to be required to elicit an ergogenic effect.

4   The most commonly used timing of caffeine supplementation is 60 minutes pre-exercise. Optimal timing of caffeine ingestion likely depends on the source of caffeine. For example, as compared to caffeine capsules, caffeine chewing gums may require a shorter waiting time from consumption to the start of the exercise session.

5   Caffeine appears to improve physical performance in both trained and untrained individuals.

6   Inter-individual differences in sport and exercise performance as well as adverse effects on sleep or feelings of anxiety following caffeine ingestion may be attributed to genetic variation associated with caffeine metabolism, and physical and psychological response. Other factors such as habitual caffeine intake may also play a role in between-individual response variation.

7   Caffeine has been shown to be ergogenic for cognitive function, including attention and vigilance, in most individuals.

8   Caffeine may improve cognitive and physical performance in some individuals under conditions of sleep deprivation.

9   The use of caffeine in conjunction with endurance exercise in the heat and at altitude is well supported when dosages range from 3–6 milligrams per kilogram and 4–6 milligrams per kilogram respectively.

10 Alternative sources of caffeine such as caffeinated chewing gum, mouth rinses, energy gels and chews have been shown to improve performance, primarily in aerobic exercise.

11 Energy drinks and pre-workout supplements containing caffeine have been demonstrated to enhance both anaerobic and aerobic performance.

So what does this mean practically?

- For shorter races of up to three hours, 3–6 milligrams per kilogram of body weight in the sixty minutes prior to the race should be sufficient to provide you with a performance impact.

- For races over three hours, there is evidence to suggest that additional top-ups throughout the duration may be beneficial. The recommendation is 1–2 milligrams per kilogram of body weight every two to four hours; however, I always encourage athletes to be mindful and adjust intake depending on how they are feeling and the environment they are running in. When working with Germain, we tend to have a Plan A when it comes to caffeine, and then he makes adjustments on race day within the parameters we know work for him through trial and testing in training.

When I work with runners, I encourage them to practise their race-day strategy. This not only means simulating fuel choices but also involves running at race paces and/or on similar terrain, if not on the actual race route. If they are going to be running at night, I encourage them to mimic this too so we can see how their body responds, especially to caffeine intake. With the feedback they provide, we then create their race strategy but always with caveats, especially around temperature and how their body is feeling in the moment.

Creatine

Another ergogenic aid that has recently received a lot of press is creatine. Creatine supplements can increase the amount of high-energy creatine phosphate stored in the muscles, and may improve performance in single or multiple sprints. They may also lead to a gain in muscle mass, which may be helpful for some athletes, depending on the sport.

As with all supplements, exceeding the maximum effective dose is not helpful. Creatine is normally found in meat and fish, but the doses used in supplementation protocols (10–20 grams per day for four or five days to load, and 2–3 grams per day for maintenance) are more than is found in normal foods. Creatine supplementation appears not to be harmful to health, but there are some things to consider:

- Muscle creatine content varies between individuals, perhaps related to gender, age or fibre type.
- There is considerable variability in the response to creatine supplementation. Individuals with the lowest initial levels, like vegetarians, female runners and older runners, show the greatest responses; and those with a resting creatine content near to the muscle threshold don't necessarily show additional enhancements.
- Thirty per cent of studies on creatine showed that individuals who consumed creatine supplements failed to achieve a worthwhile increase

in muscle creatine.
- It has been shown to enhance performance of exercise involving repeated sprints or bouts of high-intensity exercise separated by short recovery intervals, so may not be useful in all types of running.
- Although there are positive results with acute loading protocols, it seems that chronic creatine use to promote superior training adaptations may offer the greatest benefits.

The most common source of supplementation is creatine monohydrate. Studies have shown that consuming creatine doses with a substantial amount of carbohydrate – that is, 50–100 grams – enhances creatine uptake into the muscles. There appears to be no benefit in taking high doses of creatine beyond the recommendations.

A final note of caution, especially for elite and professional athletes: always be careful of any additional supplementation due to risks around anti-doping.

Collagen

Running, like all training, puts a huge amount of stress on the body and particularly on connective tissue. Strength, power and speed are directly dependent on having stiff connective tissue – that is, tendons and ligaments. However, while stiff connective tissue benefits performance, it is also associated with higher rates of injury.

The stiffness of connective tissue is dependent on two main components – collagen content and the number of cross-links within the collagen. This is another reason why we need to be mindful of how we progress with training, to prevent potential connective tissue injury.

Collagen is the most abundant protein in the human body. It is made up of amino acids, proline, hydroxyproline and glycine. Collagen provides structure to many tissues, including bones, tendons, ligaments and skin, and is essential for maintaining healthy connective tissue.

Supplements come in many forms from bovine, marine and now also plant sources, but care needs to be taken when choosing an appropriate product. Bovine collagen is the most beneficial for runners, due to the fact that it contains type I and type III collagen, which are associated with benefits to bones and muscles. Marine collagen only contains type I, which is mainly beneficial for hair, skin and nails. Presently, there are no plant-based collagen supplements that meet the right dose to support hair, skin, nails or connective tissue.

Do we need to take collagen?
Several studies have shown the potential benefits of taking a collagen supplement, especially in certain situations.

Joint health
Collagen supplements have been shown to support joint health by improving the condition of the cartilage and thus reducing stiffness and joint pain. It is well documented that our collagen levels decrease as we age and thus older runners are likely to benefit from taking a high-dose supplement. Doses of 10–15 grams of bovine collagen per day are recommended. Similarly, taking a supplement of 10 grams a day of bovine collagen may be of benefit when we are in periods of high training volume.

Connective tissue injury
Unlike muscle, connective tissue cells respond well to exercise. You only need five to ten minutes of activity to get maximal gains. You then need to wait six hours before the tissue becomes responsive again.

A study in 2017 demonstrated that an injured Major League Baseball player recovered quickly by exercising for ten minutes three times a day with six-hour intervals.[20] The study also suggested that recovery was enhanced by the addition of gelatine (which has a high concentration of collagen) consumed with vitamin C thirty to sixty minutes prior to exercise.

In my own practice, when I work with runners who present with a connective tissue or bone stress injury, I would advise the following protocol:
- Take 15–25 grams of gelatine or hydrolysed collagen with 50 milligrams of vitamin C forty to sixty minutes pre-training or rehab.

Then, once a physio has given the green light to proceed with loading, the following process has been shown to enhance recovery:
- Skipping or similar plyometric-based work (once we are confident the tendon can cope with the load) for ten to fifteen minutes three times per day with six hours in between sessions, taking 15 grams of collagen thirty to sixty minutes prior to each bout of exercise.

Bone health
Collagen supplementation has been associated with stimulating the production of bone cells, increasing bone mineral density and reducing the risk of fractures in postmenopausal women.[21] Maintaining optimal bone health is

dependent on a number of factors, including sufficient energy availability, good hormonal levels (oestrogen in females and testosterone in males), vitamin D, vitamin K, calcium and inclusion of weight-bearing exercise.

In postmenopausal women where oestrogen levels have significantly declined, there is an increased risk of reduced bone health and thus potential fractures. Hormone replacement therapy helps to mitigate some risk, but taking a collagen supplement over a twelve-month period has been shown to increase bone density significantly.[22] Benefits appear to occur with a daily intake of 5 grams of collagen. In my own practice, I tend to recommend 5 grams of collagen in the morning thirty minutes prior to any activity and then 5 grams before bed for optimal results.

More recently, using this data from studies on postmenopausal women, I have also started recommending collagen supplementation alongside improving hormonal health and energy availability to individuals who present in my clinic with very low bone density.

Beetroot juice

I remember first reading about the potential ergogenic abilities of beetroot juice when I was studying for my postgraduate qualification in applied sports nutrition in 2010. I subsequently wrote an assignment on it. It appears to be one of the few supplements that has stood the test of time, with many runners still swearing by its use. But does the science stack up?

Andrew Jones from the University of Exeter carried out some of the first studies on the impact of beetroot juice on athletic performance. He hypothesised that the high nitrate content of beetroot juice reduced time to exhaustion, allowing endurance athletes to perform at a moderate to high intensity for longer. Since then, numerous studies have shown some potential benefits to using beetroot juice for running performance, but like most research, an equal number have reported contradictions.

As with most supplements, training age, running duration and dose need to be considered before use. From a professional point of view, my advice if you are new to running is to do everything you can to get the basic fundamentals of fuelling right first, and only then think about adding something new to the mix.

For those of you who have a high training age and feel like you have hit a plateau with your progression, if you are tackling an endurance event such as a marathon there may be some benefits to taking 6–8 millimoles of nitrate in the form of beetroot juice for fifteen days leading up to the event. The timing of consumption is also key, as it appears that the nitrate concentration is optimal about 150 minutes into a run. Sadly, there is a financial implication to the dose. While eating beetroot may have some benefits, it will be impossible to know what you have consumed to ensure ergogenic properties.

Something else to be aware of is that caffeine consumption has been shown to have a negative effect on the use of beetroot juice, and there are no benefits of supplementing with beetroot juice at altitude.

CherryActive®

Another contender in the mix of potential aids to performance is a product called CherryActive®, although other brands such as Healthspan Elite have brought out their own Informed Sport-accredited, batch-tested versions for elite and professional athletes.

In essence, CherryActive® is a supplement made from tart Montmorency cherries which have a very high concentration of anthocyanin, a powerful antioxidant. Consequently, CherryActive® has become a hugely popular supplement for runners, as it has been shown to have not only anti-inflammatory properties but also high levels of melatonin that help to induce sleep and thus aid recovery.

Studies have shown that taking 1 fluid ounce of CherryActive® diluted in water thirty minutes before bed can aid sleep. Additionally, taking 1 fluid ounce of CherryActive® twice a day for five days prior to an endurance event, on the day of the event and for two days afterwards can reduce inflammation, prevent muscle damage and encourage fast recovery. This is a protocol I recommend to many runners I work with before their A races.

Sports mixes

A supplement is doing the rounds at the moment, with many fitness and run-fluencers promoting its benefits. The company behind the product reports that with its mix of minerals and vitamins, it helps with energy, immunity, gut health, hormonal and neural support, and healthy ageing.

In my opinion, with the plethora of ingredients in this product, it's tough to determine if they synchronously work to be that effective. Research can be found on the benefits of individual ingredients but not on the entire blend, and there is concern that some of the nutrients included may be contraindicated with certain medications, and the palatability of this product is also questionable.

Professionally, this is not something I would recommend. Supplements like these may be touted as an easy way to hit your micronutrient requirements, but can't override the benefits of real food.

Meal replacement drinks

These are becoming a very popular trend. Buoyed by celebrity endorsements, many individuals are turning to meal replacement drinks before, after and even during their runs as a source of nutrition. While I have no real objection to them, I do think it's a real shame that runners are choosing this over real food.

While I appreciate that many of these products are marketed as 'complete' and are fortified with vitamins and minerals, they also appear to contain a huge list of ingredients, some of which are unknown even to me. I do understand that at times we need convenience, but in my professional opinion it is always best to use real food for both fuelling and recovery. A 500-millilitre bottle of chocolate milk and a banana is still a better choice than a meal replacement drink that often contains ingredients that are not easily absorbed or digested by the human body.

CHAPTER 5

An A to Z of foods

When I first discussed the outline and framework of this book with my friend and editor Kirsty, one of the things I was really keen on was creating an A to Z of foods that all runners should be aware of. I also wanted to write a book that was accessible to everyone and didn't include products, recipes and ingredients that were not affordable or easy to find.

The cost-of-living crisis is impacting us all. We are all having to make tweaks where we can to ensure that we can live within our means. Priorities have changed, but we are also aware that certain corners should not be cut as they can have health consequences. Dietary intake is one of these key areas which we all want to prioritise, but sometimes it can feel like the area we have to compromise on the most.

Contrary to what we hear, there are many ways to maintain a healthy diet while on a budget: using frozen fruit and vegetables, stocking up on store cupboard ingredients like couscous and wholegrain pasta, and leaning towards tinned products for our protein sources, such as tuna, mackerel and beans.

As we have seen, there is a lot to take into consideration when it comes to running and eating. There are also a lot of gimmicks and trends that promise the earth but are in reality just a huge marketing ploy.

So here it is. While the list is by no means exhaustive, I have tried to pull together foods that are not only budget friendly but also provide both health and performance benefits, along with some practical tips on how to include them in your diet.

A is for ... Apples

How does the saying go? 'An apple a day keeps the doctor away!' This is not too far from the truth. Apples have numerous health benefits, but one of the key benefits to runners is the high level of quercetin, which is an antioxidant and has been demonstrated to reduce oxidative stress.

While apples don't deliver much energy for those of us who are running, they are available all year round in numerous varieties, are easy to transport and can contribute to one of our five a day.

TOP NUTRITION TIP: chop up a mix of eating and cooking apples (keep a look out for individuals who offer a free source from their apple trees, especially in autumn) and place in a pan. Add a small amount of water to the bottom of the pan, a squeeze of honey and a heaped teaspoon of mixed spice (adjust for personal preference). Cook over a low heat until the apples are stewed. They can now be added to porridge on cold mornings, or combined with Greek yoghurt and topped with granola for a recovery option post-run.

B is for ... Bread

I love bread. It is a staple in my diet and is consumed on a daily basis. However, it has had a lot of bad press in recent years, with many runners I work with being quite fearful of eating it.

Just for the record, while I love freshly baked artisan bread, I definitely can't afford this regularly and I have no issue with eating supermarket bread. Contrary to all the scaremongering about supermarket bread being an ultra-processed food (UPF), it can actually be a nutritious addition to your diet, especially if you choose wholegrain or seeded varieties. That said, even white sliced bread, although not my preferred choice, is fortified with calcium, which can be hugely beneficial to individuals who can't afford a lot of nutrient-dense food choices.

An analysis of three large US prospective cohorts, a systematic review and a meta-analysis of the prospective cohort studies looked at 'ultra-processed foods' and the associated risks of cardiovascular disease. They found that sugar and artificially sweetened drinks and processed meats were associated with a higher risk of cardiovascular disease. However, other foods labelled as UPFs, namely supermarket bread, cereals and dairy yoghurt, had an inverse association with cardiovascular disease.[23]

TOP NUTRITION TIP: bread is so versatile. It can be toasted and topped with a variety of nutrient-dense options, and a big favourite of mine is baked beans. Try this alternative option as a great pre- or post-running meal:

BAKED BEANS ON TOAST
Oil
Cumin seeds
Vegetables (fresh or frozen; my go-to are broccoli, courgettes and peppers)
Tin of baked beans (small for one person, large for two people)
Sriracha sauce
Two slices of bread
Butter

- In a small pan, heat some oil and add a handful of cumin seeds. Fry them until you get an aroma.
- Add a mix of vegetables and stir fry until they are tender, and then add a tin of baked beans.
- Add a splash of sriracha sauce and serve on two slices of buttered toast.

C is for ... Chickpeas

Although I've singled out chickpeas, in reality all tinned beans (haricot beans, black beans, black-eyed beans, kidney beans or butter beans) are a great addition to the store cupboard. It just so happens that chickpeas are one of my favourites.

A bean is a seed from several plants in the legume family. This is why the terms 'beans', 'pulses' and 'legumes' are often interchangeable. The humble bean is not only easy on the wallet but also incredibly versatile and high in nutrient density.

A portion (165 grams) of cooked chickpeas provides you with 45 grams of carbohydrate, 14.5 grams of protein, 12.5 grams of fibre, 71% of your recommended daily allowance of folate and 26% of your iron, making it an ideal option for those of us who run.

In fact, recent evidence has shown that a plant-based diet can improve carbohydrate intake in runners, and in turn improve performance. Beans also provide a high soluble fibre content, which not only supports our gut microbiome but also has been shown to reduce the risk of cardiovascular disease.

However, one piece of advice for those who are new to beans is to introduce them gradually. As previously stated, they are a source of fibre, and while this is a very important component of our diet, it can take time for digestive systems to adapt, especially if they have previously been low in fibre. In the first instance, I would definitely recommend including beans as a recovery choice over fuelling to prevent any gastrointestinal distress, especially ahead of high-intensity running such as sessions or races. That said, as a vegetarian who was brought up on a diet high in beans and pulses, I can include them throughout the day without too many gastrointestinal issues when I'm out running!

TOP NUTRITION TIP: it will be no surprise to many of you that I love curry. Growing up, it was a daily staple, and one of my go-to comfort meals is chickpea curry, perfect after a long run or fuelling ahead of a key session.

CHICKPEA CURRY

Oil
1 clove of garlic, finely chopped
1 fresh chilli, finely chopped
Thumb-sized piece of ginger, finely chopped
1 dessertspoon of cumin seeds
Tin of tomatoes
Pinch of salt
Pinch of turmeric
½ teaspoon of garam masala
Tin of chickpeas, drained
2–3 carrots, peeled and chopped
Broccoli florets

- Fry the garlic, chilli and ginger on a low heat until lightly browned.
- In a separate pan, dry fry the cumin seeds until you get an aroma.
- To the garlic add the tinned tomatoes, salt, turmeric, garam masala and cumin seeds.
- Let the tomatoes pulp down so you have an almost smooth paste which has darkened in colour.

- Add the remaining ingredients and simmer on a low heat for about 30–40 minutes until the vegetables are tender.
- Serve with rice or naan bread, Greek yoghurt and mango chutney.

D is for ... Dairy

Dairy is definitely one of those food groups that creates great controversy, especially around animal welfare and environmental implications. I value these concerns, but professionally, dairy is still one of the most nutrient-dense food groups that is beneficial to health.

During childhood, we are constantly told about the benefits of dairy for our bone health. Indeed, these benefits continue into adulthood, especially as bone density starts to decline from our late twenties. I recommend that all athletes aim for three or four servings a day, which provides 1,000–1,200 milligrams of calcium.

It has been well documented that milk is the ideal choice for recovery after exercise.[24] Sports nutrition recommendations for optimal recovery suggest ingestion of both carbohydrate and protein, in a 3:1 ratio respectively. This ratio has proven to be the most effective at replenishing glycogen stores after high-intensity or long endurance training, when these stores will be completely or almost completely depleted.

Additionally, milk is a good source of minerals and electrolytes, making it an ideal choice for rehydrating. While there are many plant drink substitutes, none can provide this 3:1 ratio, with chocolate soya milk probably being the closest possible alternative.

Yoghurt is also a great recovery option. I particularly favour Greek yoghurt, due to its very high protein content. Most natural Greek yoghurt provides 10 grams of protein per 100 grams, which is double the amount in standard yoghurts. Protein is an important nutrient required in the response to exercise in order to repair and rebuild muscles, helping them to adapt to the training process.

Many of us worry about eating cheese due to its high fat content. However, not only does it provide us with calcium and magnesium but it is also one of the only foods providing us with phosphorus. All three of these are essential nutrients required for bone health. Recent studies also confirmed that the saturated fatty acids found in cheese appear to have protective benefits for our cardiovascular health.

TOP NUTRITION TIP: if you are worried about eating cheese, keep portions to around the size of a small matchbox. Crumble some feta cheese with half an avocado, add lemon and chilli flakes and mash together to make a refreshing dip or topping for your toast or baked potato.

E is for ... Eggs

They may be small, but eggs really pack a punch when it comes to nutritional value. Two medium eggs provide around 12–15 grams of protein and 100% of our daily requirement of vitamin B12, which is essential for the formation of red blood cells as well as being packed with selenium, a powerful antioxidant. This makes eggs ideal as a recovery food post-training.

A lot of people still avoid eggs due to concerns over cholesterol, but in fact a medium egg only contains 4.6 grams of fat, of which only 1.3 grams comes from saturated fat. And if you still need convincing, studies have shown that people who consumed two eggs for breakfast every morning had better glycaemic control later in the day, preventing energy dips and managing appetite.[25]

TOP NUTRITION TIP: try making a frittata – load it up with vegetables, throw in a handful of feta cheese or tofu to ensure you meet your calcium requirements for the day and serve with wholemeal pitta for an easy but nutrient-dense recovery meal.

F is for ... Fish

While all fish is beneficial to runners as it provides a great source of protein, oily fish is one of the best sources of omega-3 fatty acids. These are essential fatty acids and their benefits have been recognised on the nutrition circuit for some time. The three main and most researched types are EPA (eicosapentaenoic acid), DHA (docosahexaenoic acid) and ALA (alpha-linolenic acid). There is no doubt that runners should be looking to include omega-3 fatty acids within their diet. The health benefits alone, particularly with regard to cardiovascular health and reducing inflammation, are strong and robust. More recently, research has been showing strong positive associations with prevention of cognitive decline.

Although the evidence may be more limited and further research is still required, the specific benefits linked to exercise provide even more reason to ensure appropriate dietary intake. These include positive associations with an improved inflammatory response to exercise, a reduction in muscle soreness, enhanced muscular recovery and a decreased risk of injury. Additionally, omega-3 fatty acids have been shown to encourage bronchodilation, thus supporting lung function, essential for most runners. As a vegetarian, I don't eat fish but this is one of the key reasons why I take omega-3 fatty acid supplements to support and help manage my sarcoidosis.

As with most nutrients, a food-first approach is always the best policy. The inclusion of oily fish at least twice a week would be the most appropriate, with fresh salmon, sardines and bluefin tuna being the best sources. Tinned versions of these oily fish still have benefits – the doses are slightly lower but they are kinder to the wallet. The exception is tinned tuna, where a lot of valuable EPA and DHA is lost due to processing.

For runners who do not consume oily fish, a supplement can be useful, with plant-based runners choosing an algae-based option. The recommended dosage with regard to supplementation will vary a little based on activity level and the type of sport, but for runners, aiming for 0.5–2 grams of EPA and DHA combined daily seems to be appropriate.

TOP NUTRITION TIP: try this recipe for smoked mackerel pâté, which makes one large pot with around two servings.

SMOKED MACKEREL PÂTÉ

2 smoked mackerel fillets
60 grams of cream cheese
Juice of half a lemon

- Remove the skin from the fillets and flake the fillets into a large bowl. Add the cream cheese and lemon juice.
- Blend until a pâté- or dip-like consistency.
- Serve with oatcakes or toast for a recovery snack; or, for a more substantial recovery meal, try it with baked sweet potato.

G is for ... Grains

Grains are the edible seeds of plants in the cereal family, such as wheat, rice, corn, oats and barley. They are a vital part of many cultures' diets and are a good source of fibre, vitamins and minerals.

Grains are divided into two categories: wholegrains and refined grains.

Wholegrains contain the entire grain kernel, including the bran, germ and endosperm. Examples include brown rice, wholegrain pasta and bread. Refined grains have been milled to remove the bran and germ, which improves their texture and shelf life but also removes some nutrients. Refined grains are often enriched with some nutrients that were lost during processing, such as B vitamins, but not fibre. Examples include white rice, white pasta and white flour.

Wholegrains are generally considered more nutritious than refined grains and have been linked to health benefits such as a lower risk of heart disease and diabetes. However, while refined grains have been associated with negative health outcomes, there is little robust evidence for this and most of the claims have been observational.

While we all need to be mindful of consuming foods that are made with refined grains, such as biscuits, cakes and pastries, there is no evidence to restrict foods like white rice, pasta and crumpets that can actually be very beneficial to a runner's diet. In certain scenarios, such as prior to race day or ahead of a high-intensity training session, it is more advantageous to consume refined grains such as white rice, white flour-based products and pasta, as they are more easily absorbed and can deliver energy quickly to the working muscles.

TOP NUTRITION TIP: try serving this amazing aubergine curry with white rice or pitta breads ahead of a long run or higher-intensity training session.

AUBERGINE CURRY (MEAT EATERS CAN ADD SOME CHICKEN FOR ADDED PROTEIN)

2 aubergines
1 onion
Oil
Small pieces of fresh ginger, crushed
1 clove of garlic
Large tin of chopped tomatoes
1 large tomato, chopped
¼ teaspoon of salt
½ teaspoon of garam masala
¼ teaspoon of chilli powder

- Place two aubergines under the grill. Keep turning them and let them cook all the way through – the skin will go all crispy. Once they are cooked, leave to cool.
- In the meantime, dice an onion and add it to some hot oil in a wok, balti pan or deep frying pan. Add some crushed ginger and a glove of garlic.
- Cook these three over a very low heat. Keep turning until they are golden brown (beyond the translucent stage).
- Add a large tin of chopped tomatoes and a large fresh tomato, chopped.
- Cook all of the ingredients together until you have a fairly smooth sauce.
- Add all the spices and mix these in.
- Remove the skin from the cooled aubergine and add the pulp to the tomato sauce.
- Mix everything together and cook on a very low heat for 30–45 minutes. The longer you leave it, the better the flavour.
- Add yoghurt to serve.

H is for … Hummus

We've already discussed the nutritional benefits of chickpeas, but the combination with tahini, garlic, lemon and olive oil makes this a nutrient-packed dip full of vitamins and minerals.

The chickpeas provide soluble fibre, an important component of the diet that has been positively linked with improved heart and gut health. Chickpeas are also high in protein, iron, folate and B vitamins, making them a great choice for everyone, particularly vegetarians and vegans whose diets may be naturally low in these things. Similarly, tahini is sesame seed paste and an excellent source of calcium; this is especially important as a non-dairy option for individuals who avoid or cannot tolerate dairy.

While hummus is often associated with being high in fat, it is usually made with olive oil or rapeseed oil. Both are good sources of unsaturated fatty acids, which should be making up the majority of our overall fat intake.

Hummus is very versatile – it can be used as a sandwich filling, a jacket potato topping or a dip to be eaten with vegetables, and is perfect as a high-protein snack between meals.

TOP NUTRITION TIP: for a great recovery lunch, grill a mix of Mediterranean-style vegetables such as courgettes, peppers, aubergines and tomatoes. Place these over two slices of toasted sourdough and top with a generous serving of hummus.

I is for ... Ice cream

While this is not necessarily top of the nutritional choices, it is important to appreciate that true healthy eating is actually about balance; while you should aim to make your diet nutrient-dense for the majority of the time, there is still room for the occasional less-nutrient-dense option.

If you have been training or racing in very hot climates, having ice cream as part of your recovery protocol can help to bring about an initial cooling effect (although the higher fat content of ice cream does mean that the body takes more time to digest and this actually slightly raises your temperature in the long run). The high sugar content is useful in starting to replace depleted glycogen stores. So while this isn't the number-one choice for recovery, there is a time and place when it can be consumed.

TOP NUTRITION TIP: one way to make ice cream a little more nutrient-dense is to add it to your recovery shake – blend a banana, milk and a scoop of vanilla ice cream as an option post-high-intensity training session.

J is for ... Jelly

Again, this may seem controversial, but work with me!

During high-intensity exercise of more than forty-five minutes, or more moderate-intensity endurance training over ninety minutes, it is recommended that we take on fuel in the form of carbohydrates to spare our glycogen stores, and enable the ability to maintain our pace and intensity. The general guidelines are to take on around 40–60 grams of carbohydrate per hour, ideally starting about twenty to thirty minutes into a run (we will discuss this further in chapter 6). Remember, the harder your muscles and body are working, the quicker you will drain your glycogen stores.

There are many sport-specific products on the market, including gels, drinks and bars. I will go into more detail about these in the next chapter, but one thing that is clear is that all sports nutrition comes with a price tag. One alternative you could try is packet jelly. It is cheap, it comes in an array of flavours and each individual cube provides around 10 grams of carbohydrate. When comparing ingredients, packet jellies are fairly similar to a lot of sports nutrition products, but they cost a fraction of the price.

TOP NUTRITION TIP: prior to a race, cut a packet of jelly in half. This way you will know that each half provides you with 45 grams of carbohydrate. Remember, as with all fuel options, practise in training to ensure you can tolerate this before using it on race day.

K is for ... Kidney beans

We are returning to the legume family, and this time the spotlight is on kidney beans. These little purple jewels provide a great source of soluble fibre, iron, folate, magnesium, potassium and phosphates, which are all necessary for body processes to occur optimally. In addition, they are low in fat and reasonably high in protein, making them particularly useful to vegetarians and vegans.

The high fibre content is hugely beneficial for digestive health. Studies have shown that including a variety of beans and pulses in your diet can support your gut microbiome.

TOP NUTRITION TIP: Drain a tin of kidney beans and mix with chopped pepper, tomato, coriander, a squeeze of lime and chilli flakes for a nutrient-dense filling for a wholemeal pitta or wrap.

L is for ... Lentils

Growing up, dhal was an absolute staple in my diet. I remember the jars on our kitchen shelf full of different coloured varieties of lentils: green, red, yellow split pea and black.

Like beans, lentils are an excellent cheap source of protein, but they are even more versatile and can often be added to dishes as a meat replacement. Why not try boiling up some red lentils and supplementing half the mince in a bolognese sauce with them? Similarly, they make a great addition to salads for a hearty and nutritious lunch. In addition, lentils are high in iron, high in fibre and low in fat.

Some dry versions will need soaking overnight before cooking, or equally you can use a pressure cooker, tinned or even packet varieties.

TOP NUTRITION TIP: this was one of my favourite dhal recipes growing up. It does take a bit of time to make but it is worth it and can also be frozen, so it is useful for another meal when time is short.

THREE-LENTIL DHAL

Oil
2 cloves of garlic
1 large piece of fresh ginger
¾ mug red lentils, washed
¾ mug yellow split peas, soaked overnight
¾ mug black lentils, soaked overnight
1 large onion, chopped
Tin of tomatoes
½ teaspoon of salt
¾ teaspoon of garam masala
Chilli powder to personal preference
Frozen or fresh coriander

- In a large saucepan, add oil and cook the garlic and ginger until they are golden brown.
- Add the three types of lentils to the pan with five mugs of water.
- Bring to the boil and then simmer until the lentils are blended and you get a more puréed consistency.
- In a small frying pan, cook the onion. Once translucent, add the tin of tomatoes, ½ teaspoon of salt, ¾ teaspoon of garam masala and chilli powder to personal preference.
- Let the tomato sauce cook until reduced and quite thick, and then add to the lentil pan.
- Cook on a low heat and allow all the ingredients to merge and blend.
- Top with coriander.
- Serve with rice or pittas or chapatis and natural yoghurt.

M is for ... Macaroni

While I'm using macaroni as my chosen example, I'm really talking about pasta in general. It just so happened that macaroni worked with my alphabetical shopping list!

For years, pasta has been known as the endurance fuel of choice. However, in recent years, many athletes have been persuaded to go gluten-free, with no real evidence or performance rationale. Pasta, particularly white pasta, has become associated with being a processed food (see the earlier point about refined grains on page 82) and something that should be avoided. But can something that is made simply from wheat and egg be bad for us?

Pasta is a great source of carbohydrate, which is necessary for our bodies to work at a high intensity, or over a long duration. It also provides B vitamins, folate and thiamine, which are necessary for many biological processes within the body. Wholegrain varieties have the additional benefit of providing fibre, which is important for our gut microbiome.

When it comes to whether white or wholegrain pasta is best, it comes down to preference – both are nutrient-dense, and can be beneficial in different scenarios. I personally tend to recommend white pasta before runs and wholegrain pasta after.

TOP NUTRITION TIP: serve with pesto and roasted vegetables, topped with a protein source of your choice.

N is for ... Nut butter

Most runners are surprised when I mention they can eat nut butter. Yes, it is high in fat, but it is high in good fats and provides you with so many other essential nutrients, such as calcium, iron, magnesium, phosphorus and vitamin E. In addition to fatty acids, nuts and nut butters are a protein source, which makes them useful components for vegan and vegetarian diets.

One thing to watch, though: they aren't such a good choice after a high-intensity training session, as the fat content slows down the absorption of protein needed for recovery. One way round this is to have a glass of milk first (soya if you are vegan) and follow it with your toast and nut butter. Whether you choose peanut, almond, cashew or hazelnut is down to personal preference. Peanut butter tends to be my staple and I generally choose brands that don't have added sugar or palm oil.

TOP NUTRITION TIP: I can eat peanut butter at pretty much any time of the day, and even straight out of the pot, but you may like this recipe as a mid-afternoon snack or even as an after-dinner dessert option.

POTTED 'GREEK' CAKE (SERVES 1)
Nut butter of your choice
100 grams of plain Greek/Greek-style yoghurt
Berry compote (see page 61)
Honey
Fresh berries to serve (optional)

- Put 1 dessertspoon of nut butter of your choice in the bottom of a ramekin or similar-sized bowl or tea cup.
- Separately mix the yoghurt with a generous serving of berry compote and a heaped teaspoon of honey.
- Place the yoghurt mix on top of the nut butter. Top with a couple of fresh berries if you fancy, and either chill in the fridge until ready to serve or eat immediately.

O is for ... Oats

I'm pretty sure that if I asked most runners for their number one store cupboard ingredient, oats would win a high percentage of the vote. It is well documented that porridge is one of the best breakfast options to start the day. It is low in fat, high in soluble fibre and a great source of complex carbohydrate. This means that it releases energy slowly throughout the day, preventing blood sugar fluctuations or energy crashes.

That said, I appreciate that not everyone is a porridge fan and here is the beauty: oats are hugely versatile and don't necessarily need to be eaten as porridge for you to get nutritional benefits. You can eat oats uncooked in the form of overnight oats or standard muesli or, if you are feeling particularly creative, why not try oaty pancakes?

If you really are not a morning oat person, you could have oatcakes or even make your own energy bars or flapjacks, which are ideal as a training snack or before an early morning run. Whichever way, they should definitely be on your list as a go-to food to fuel your running endeavours.

TOP NUTRITION TIP: try adding oats to a morning smoothie for a portable breakfast option – it works well when blended with milk, banana and honey.

P is for ... Potatoes

Baked, mashed, boiled, roasted ... the potato is one of my favourite carbohydrate choices at mealtimes. Potatoes are nutrient-rich, especially if you eat the skins, which provide both fibre and a high concentration of vitamin C. They can also be alternated with sweet potatoes, which offer a slightly different taste and texture, plus are high in beta-carotene, an important antioxidant. Both provide slow-release energy, making them ideal fuel options before or after exercise.

They are perfect just baked and served with oily fish as a recovery meal or added to a risotto for a pre-endurance training meal. They can be added to salads, and sweet potatoes in particular make fabulous soups for lunchtime options, helping to prevent that 4 p.m. sugar slump. I am also partial to salted roasted potatoes during a long ultrarun.

TOP NUTRITION TIP: good potato options pre-run include:
- Large sweet potato baked and served with roasted Mediterranean vegetables (peppers – the more colours, the more vitamins – mushrooms, courgette, aubergine, red onion and garlic roasted in a small amount of olive oil) and topped with a generous helping of feta cheese. The focus here is on fuelling the body with carbohydrates, but the feta adds a tang to the sweetness of the potato and provides essential bone-building calcium and phosphorus.
- Large jacket potato with hummus and beetroot salad (raw beetroot grated, salad leaves, cucumber, tomatoes and grated carrots) with a coriander and lime salad dressing.

Another favourite potato topping of mine is carrot and cumin:
- Grate a couple of carrots.
- In a small frying pan, heat some oil and add a generous handful of cumin seeds.
- Once you can smell the cumin, add the grated carrot, a pinch of salt and chilli flakes.
- Mix thoroughly and serve with your potato and hummus.

For good recovery meals, try these ideas:
- Medium jacket potato with chilli. Try substituting half your normal mince with red lentils, which will still provide you with muscle-recovering protein but with less overall fat. Lentils also provide soluble fibre, which will help to control blood sugars. This meal is also rich in iron.
- Large sweet potato with smoked mackerel pâté. Try blending two smoked mackerel fillets with two tablespoons of 0% fat Greek yoghurt, the juice of half a lemon and a dash of horseradish; you can also substitute the yoghurt with low-fat cream cheese if you prefer. This makes a perfect recovery meal – it is big on protein, with anti-inflammatory omega-3 fats to aid muscle recovery.

Q is for ... Quinoa

Quinoa is a nutrient-dense gluten-free grain. It is the only grain that contains all nine essential amino acids and thus is very popular and useful in vegan and vegetarian diets, not only as a carbohydrate source but also as protein. Additionally, it is a great source of magnesium and zinc, which are necessary for optimal muscle contraction and repair.

Quinoa is a very versatile ingredient: it can be added to curries as a bulking agent, served as a side dish to accompany a casserole or used as an integral component of a salad.

TOP NUTRITION TIP: try making a large quantity of quinoa at the start of the week and add different components every day to provide yourself with nutrient-dense lunch options.

R is for ... Rice

Did you know that rice is a complex carbohydrate that provides a primary source of energy for more than half of the world's population? It is naturally gluten-free and contains many essential vitamins and minerals, including B vitamins, potassium, magnesium, selenium, fibre, iron and zinc.

As with pasta, whether you choose white or brown is usually a personal preference, but generally I would suggest white rice before running, particularly if it is your carbohydrate choice in the few days ahead of a race.

Brown rice is a definite favourite in my household – we eat it several days a week either with a curry or stir fry, or as a type of pilaf with vegetables and black beans.

TOP NUTRITION TIP: I recently made this curry for some good friends when they came over for dinner. I had made it for Ewen and me before, but it was the first time I had shared it with anyone else. They gave it the thumbs-up, so I thought I would add it to the book.

KERALAN TOFU CURRY

2 cloves of garlic
Thumb-sized piece of ginger
1 chilli
Oil
Vegetables of your choice
Tofu – 1 pack (160g) of marinated pieces
Tin of kidney beans (drained)
Cumin seeds
Pinch of salt
¾ teaspoon of garam masala
400–600ml coconut milk (1–1.5 tins)

- Finely chop the garlic, ginger and deseeded chilli.
- Fry gently in oil on a low heat until the ginger and garlic are lightly browned.
- Add any vegetables you want, plus the tofu and kidney beans.
- In a frying pan, dry-fry some cumin seeds.
- Once the vegetables are slightly cooked, add the cumin seeds, a pinch of salt and the garam masala.
- Add the coconut milk and simmer gently for about 45 minutes.
- Serve with rice.

S is for ... Seeds

Seeds may be small but they are jam-packed with high nutrient value. Flax, sunflower, sesame, chia and linseeds all have a place, providing many benefits. Flaxseeds and linseeds are useful sources of omega-3 fatty acids for vegetarians, vegans or individuals who do not consume oily fish. They are high in ALA (alpha-linolenic acid), which can be converted to DHA (docosahexaenoic acid) in the body, although the process is not very efficient.

All seeds are high in fibre and thus useful to support our gut microbiome, but contrary to popular trends you don't need to part with your hard-earned cash and buy a branded product that deems itself superior. Blending your own mix is just as nutritious at a fraction of the price.

TOP NUTRITION TIP: try toasting sunflower seeds and adding them to roasted vegetables for a nuttier taste and texture. Grind up some flaxseeds and add a daily tablespoon to porridge or smoothies for a great start to the day; or try mixing flaxseed oil into mashed potato to make it more nutrient-dense and give it a nutty flavour.

T is for ... Tofu

Tofu is a must-have for all vegan and vegetarian diets as it is one of the only plant-based sources of protein that contains all the essential amino acids. It is also a great source of calcium, supporting bone health and muscle contraction.

While some people may struggle with its blandness, tofu is hugely versatile as it takes on the flavour of whatever you are cooking. Failing that, you can always marinate it prior to cooking. For those who want an even simpler life, there are now many varieties available, including smoked, or flavoured with basil or olives. These can be eaten hot or cold as a snack or meal. Try eating tofu in stir fries or curries as a meat alternative, thrown into a salad, or simply served with salad in a pitta pocket as an alternative to sandwiches at lunchtime.

TOP NUTRITION TIP: Ewen makes a great tofu stir fry which is so good we tend to eat it at least once if not twice a week. The key is probably in the fresh herbs.

CHILLI TOFU STIR FRY

Thumb-sized piece of ginger
1 clove of garlic
1 chilli
Oil
Tofu – 1 pack (160g) of marinated pieces
Vegetables of your choice, such as peppers, broccoli, courgettes or mini corn
Soy sauce, sriracha sauce and honey (mix to your personal preference)
Rice or noodles

- Finely chop and fry the fresh ginger, garlic and chilli in a wok with some oil.
- Add the tofu as this gives it a firmer texture. We use the marinated version, but you can use plain or smoked – all types work.
- Once the tofu has taken on some colour, add the vegetables.
- Stir fry for 5–7 minutes and then add a good helping of soy sauce, sriracha sauce and a squirt of honey.
- Serve with rice or noodles.

U is for ... Udon noodles

Udon are chewy Japanese noodles made from wheat flour, water and salt, typically served in soups and broths. Unlike buckwheat soba noodles, they are not gluten-free but are slightly thicker in texture. They are paler in colour than ramen noodles and tend to be subtle in taste. One of the most important things to note about udon noodles (unlike ramen) is that they are not made with egg, making them a great choice for vegan runners.

All noodle options make a great alternative to rice, pasta, potato or grains as a carbohydrate source for any meal.

TOP NUTRITION TIP: noodles are another food that can also be useful during long ultra events, as long as you have a crew that can make them for you. I recently suggested Damian try them made with a vegetable stock cube, keeping some of the liquid and adding soy sauce and sweet chilli sauce for another savoury fuelling option. He gave them the thumbs-up!

V is for ... Vegetable oil

There is so much controversy over what to cook with – coconut oil, olive oil or even butter. For every article that suggests one option, another article slams it, and it can be difficult to know what you really should use to cook with.

As with most things, eating an excess will not be beneficial to health. Presently, the favoured recommendation is to keep saturated fat to a minimum, with the exception of saturated fat from dairy, that is milk, cheese and yoghurt. This doesn't mean that you can never eat butter or coconut oil, but it does suggest that they should not be your preferred choice for all cooking.

In particular, coconut oil is high in medium chain triglycerides (MCT). Our bodies can only absorb 30 grams of MCT a day. A few years ago, I worked with a lady who was a runner. She came to see me as she was having real issues with her digestive system, especially when running. After our assessment, it was clear that she had swapped all fat intake to be coconut, which was the big nutrition trend at the time. We reduced her intake of coconut oil and replaced it with a mix including some butter, vegetable and olive oils, and all her digestive issues cleared up within a few days.

Vegetable oil has had its own bad press in the past, which was not and is still not warranted. What most people don't appreciate is that vegetable oil is actually 100% rapeseed oil in the UK. Rapeseed is highly nutritious, low in saturated fat, budget friendly, and doesn't change in structure or stability when heated to high temperatures, thus making it a great choice for daily cooking.

TOP NUTRITION TIP: I use vegetable oil for all my cooking, and here is another recipe that you may enjoy.

THREE-BEAN CHILLI

Vegetable oil
1 clove of garlic, chopped
Thumb-sized piece of ginger, chopped
1 dessertspoon of cumin seeds
1 red pepper, chopped
Grated carrots
1 carton of passata
Pinch of salt
Chilli flakes
1 tin of chickpeas, 1 tin of black beans and 1 tin of kidney beans
Frozen or fresh coriander

- Place the oil in a large pan or wok, and add the garlic, ginger and half of the cumin seeds.
- As soon as it becomes aromatic, add the red pepper and grated carrots and allow to cook until tender.
- Add the passata, salt, chilli flakes and the rest of the cumin seeds.
- Mix in the drained beans and coriander, and allow to simmer for about 10 minutes.
- Serve with your carbohydrate of choice.

W is for ... Walnuts

Walnuts are another great plant source of omega-3 fatty acids, particularly ALA (alpha-linolenic acid). Additionally, they are extremely high in antioxidants, making them an excellent nutritional choice for anyone who is physically active. As previously mentioned, a number of studies have looked at the benefits of omega-3 fatty acids, which includes EPA, DHA and ALA, with strong evidence to suggest that a diet rich in omega-3 fatty acids has some protective factors against heart disease. The high antioxidant content of walnuts ensures that they contribute towards reducing oxidative stress after intense exercise.

TOP NUTRITION TIP: try toasting walnuts and then rolling them in honey to use as a nutrient-dense topping for porridge in the winter months. Alternatively, add them to banana bread, which can then be toasted and topped with honey or nut butter as a great early morning pre-run snack. Walnuts also make a great option as a base for pesto when blended with other nuts, basil leaves and olive oil.

X is for ...

There isn't one!

Y is for ... Yeast extract

Yeast extract, such as Marmite, is packed full of B vitamins. These play an essential role in the processes involved in releasing energy from food during exercise, recovery and repair, and optimal immune health. Studies have shown that active individuals who have low B vitamin levels may have a decreased ability to perform high-intensity exercise.

While yeast extract might not be everyone's favourite choice to have on toast at breakfast, it can be added to stews, bolognese and soups, not only to enrich but also to add flavour and depth.

TOP NUTRITION TIP: a few years ago, when I was working as team manager for the GB 24-hour squad, a lot of the runners wanted something that was a savoury alternative to gels but could also be easily consumed. I came up with this as an option, which a lot of them tried and continued to use into the championships:

- In a freezer bag, add mashed potato, Marmite and cheese. Cut the corner off the freezer bag or use a reusable gel container and take on as fuel.

Z is for ... Za'atar

It was always going to be hard to find a store cupboard ingredient – or any food ingredient for that matter – to start with Z. I opted for za'atar, but like previous entries above, I'm actually referring to dried herbs and spices in general.

Za'atar is a Middle Eastern herb that originates from the oregano and marjoram family but actually has the flavour of thyme and sage. It adds flavour to meat marinades, and can be added to dips or scattered over roasted vegetables. Herbs and spices such as za'atar have high antioxidant scores and properties, making them ideal to aid recovery after hard training sessions. There is evidence to suggest that a diet high in antioxidants can reduce the extent of oxidative damage following high-intensity exercise.

TOP NUTRITION TIP: try scattering za'atar leaves over hummus and tomato layered on a couple of slices of sourdough toast as a nutrient-rich recovery lunch.

CHAPTER 6

The kitchen

Nutrition can make or break your training and thus your ability to race, if that is your end goal.

In chapters 4 and 5, we went into a bit more detail about the importance of nutrition and the role it plays in fuelling and recovery. We looked at the general components of a runner's diet and discussed what foods are good to have in your store cupboard. In this chapter, we are going to go into a little more detail about training, looking at different distances and terrains and whether they have an impact on how to eat. We will discuss how to fuel during and around race day, and how to ensure that we are fuelling enough for life and training. We will also look at nutrient timing and how it has an integral role to play in hormonal balance, bone health and maintaining your immune system, which are key not just for health but also optimal performance. Finally, we will bring all of this together practically, alongside juggling daily life, to demonstrate how a healthy runner is a happy runner!

The importance of glycogen

When it comes to running performance, I've said it many times but carbohydrate really is king. Carbohydrate gets broken down into glucose, which is the preferred currency of energy for the body and brain.

Carbohydrate is stored as glycogen within the liver and muscles. It is this source within the muscles that is the most readily available energy for working muscles, releasing energy more quickly than other sources. However, this storage facility is limited. If the muscles are inadequately fuelled, this leads to fatigue, poor performance and, in the longer term, stress and the potential for a greater risk of injury and illness.

To give you some context, it takes 400 to 500 grams of carbohydrate to have completely full muscle glycogen stores, with an additional 80 grams in liver glycogen, mainly used to maintain energy to the brain. Many of us take the brain for granted and don't appreciate that it also needs a supply of energy. In fact, our brain needs around 120–130 grams of glucose a day to work optimally.

BEHAVIOUR CHANGE/DISTRESS TOLERANCE

When I work with athletes and athletic individuals with a more complex relationship with food, most of them are very aware of their dysfunctional relationships with food and exercise, but are confused about why they can't challenge and change the behaviour. My response is that it's just not as simple as that, both psychologically and physiologically. Having an intellectual awareness of your issues is very important in order to change. However, it is also important to appreciate that all human behaviour has a purpose, and often that purpose is protection.

I spoke earlier about my experience with anorexia and how my restrictive eating and maintaining a low weight wasn't for aesthetics but provided me with a coping mechanism, an ability to shut down all the noise and hatred I felt towards myself. Often when I'm working with someone, I can help them to appreciate that there is a somatic response that is keeping them stuck, and this is where my mindfulness training comes into practice.

However, I also educate them on the amount of energy it takes to create new neural pathways and change a behaviour. I explain that if we were both to decide on the same behaviour change – let's use doing more weight sessions than running as an example – while we would both experience a term known as 'distress tolerance' due to the change, my brain would adapt to this change a lot quicker than theirs because I provide it with enough nutrition and have adequate amounts of glucose.

So not only are carbohydrates important for our active bodies but they are also really important to support our brain health.

As we covered earlier, when muscle glycogen is at full capacity, at most this will last for around 90–120 minutes' running at 65–75% of our maximal heart rate, or a perceived exertion of around six or seven out of ten. The faster our speed, the faster our stores will deplete. Therefore, if we train most days, our glycogen stores are always slightly depleted.[26]

Let's look at this in a little more detail. Firstly, what does 500 grams of carbohydrate look like? Contrary to what you might think, it is actually a lot of food. Here is an example of a typical daily intake for someone who is moderately active for around sixty to ninety minutes a day.

Breakfast
- Porridge made with 50 grams of oats and 250 millilitres of cow's milk with walnuts and 2 teaspoons of honey (58 grams of carbohydrate)

Mid-morning snack
- Packet of fruit oatcakes (five biscuits) and 300 millilitres of cow's milk latte (50 grams of carbohydrate)

Lunch
- Beans on two slices of wholemeal toast and a 200-millilitre glass of juice (88 grams of carbohydrate)

Pre-run snack
- Two crumpets with peanut butter and banana (65 grams of carbohydrate)

Evening meal within thirty minutes of finishing the run (more on this later)
- 60 grams of rice (dried weight) cooked and served with tofu stir fry (48 grams of carbohydrate)

Followed by
- 170 grams of Greek yoghurt with 40 grams of granola (32 grams of carbohydrate)

The sum total of carbohydrate is 341 grams, which does meet the requirements of 5 grams per kilogram of body weight for someone who is 68 kilograms, but is still a little off reaching the amount you would need to achieve full glycogen stores. It also explains why we have the concept of carbohydrate loading, especially before a race.

This helps us to understand the importance of refuelling in between runs or training sessions. We can then stay on top of our glycogen stores in order to prevent fatigue and injury and optimise our adaptation from the run session. If the tank is empty, even if we complete a run, we haven't got the energy in the system to allow for the cellular transcription and adaptation that needs to happen for progression.

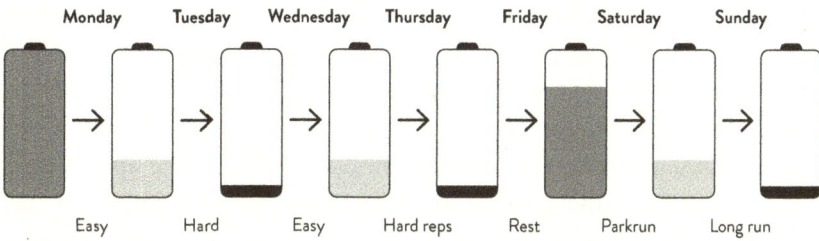

Figure 6.1

While I don't want to simplify the human body to a machine, it can be useful to look at glycogen stores a bit like a battery. Figure 6.1 demonstrates that even if we start with full glycogen stores on Monday, by the time we have completed an easy sixty-minute run, we will have depleted our stores to around a third. Even if we manage to fuel well and fill our stores up for Tuesday, if this is a hard session such as six 3-minute intervals, we will have completely depleted our stores by the end of the session.

In this way, you can see how vital it is to fuel in between runs or training sessions. If you are running a minimum of four or five times a week, those rest days are really key and definitely should not be days when you eat less. Remember that each rest day serves a purpose. It is an opportunity for your body to rest, take stock, adapt and also prepare for your next training day.

I personally find that by listening to my body and appetite, I never go too far wrong. In fact, during the build-up to a race, when my training volume is high, my appetite increases. On days when I have done a higher intensity or longer run, I struggle a little to meet my full requirements, due to the effort and time it takes for blood flow to return to the stomach, but my body always tries to catch up on rest days and I usually find this is when my hunger properly kicks in and I always respond. Post-race, once my body has recovered and I go back to more of a maintenance running programme, I'm still hungry and I still eat well, but I definitely don't find myself having quite the ferocious appetite of previous months.

One of the biggest and most concerning mistakes I see in my field of work is individuals who believe that they have to earn their food rather than fuel their training. The problem with this narrative is that it sets you up to fail. You start believing that unless you have 'moved your body' that day, you don't deserve to eat, especially when it comes to carbohydrates. We've spoken previously about all the scaremongering around carbohydrates, but I hope you can now start to see the role they play not just for energy but for your brain, hormonal health, bone health and actual progression from training. This is also why fuelling well (yes, with carbohydrates) on your rest day is important.

The confusion appears to be related to misconceptions around what happens when we consume carbohydrates and our total body glycogen stores are full. The body does indeed store this excess glucose in our adipose (fat) cells. However, contrary to popular understanding, this is a common and absolutely normal occurrence, and it does not mean you are putting down fat or going to put on weight, as it is a temporary state. In fact, fat storage and fat breakdown is in a constant state of flux. When you look around, you will very rarely see people physically change overnight or even over a few weeks. Physical change occurs over much longer periods of times (months or years) and usually involves a situation where food consumption has been taken to an extreme.

Remember that a healthy body works for you. If you look after your body, listen to it and respond to its needs, it will work for you, not against you. So instead of 'will run for cake', it should actually be 'will eat cake to run'.

CASE STUDY

A few years ago, I worked with a semi-professional marathon runner who was very much stuck in the cycle of earning her food, to the point where on special occasions like Christmas, birthdays or anniversaries, she would plan her long training run on the day of the celebration so that she felt able to eat and drink what she wanted and relax.

However, what she didn't appreciate was that by not fuelling for her runs, or even really during them, she was setting her body up to fail. In her head, this was a way of controlling her appetite and thus weight, but actually when you don't give your body enough energy around your training, not only do you prevent vital hormonal cascades that need to happen for progression in performance and body composition, but you also alter your stress and appetite hormones. This in turn results in the body switching on fat storage, and leads you to eat to excess post-training. It is the body's way of ensuring that there is enough energy in times of scarcity.

While I tried to educate her on this, she really struggled to change her mindset. She suffered a lot of setbacks in her running and sadly never quite hit her potential.

Carbohydrate loading

Carbohydrate loading is something that is usually discussed in the endurance side of running. It is probably relatable to any distance from 10 kilometres upwards.

As we have seen, when we work hard, we deplete our glycogen stores very quickly, so the aim before a hard effort or race is to have full glycogen stores. This can prove challenging on a daily basis. Before a race, training drops down in the taper and the aim is to try and take on enough carbohydrates to ensure full stores on the morning of the race day. We have seen how much food it takes to fill our glycogen stores, so this is not really something we should leave until the day before the race, let alone in the evening before. I recommend thinking about carbohydrate loading a few days before.

10 kilometres to half marathon distance

- If your race is on Saturday morning, ideally start thinking about carbohydrate intake on Wednesday and Thursday. On Friday, eat what feels most comfortable, but I usually suggest eating your main meal at lunchtime and having a lighter meal or snack in the evening to aid digestion. Don't forget to hydrate. Studies have shown that we store glycogen more efficiently if we are hydrated. I tend to suggest drinking electrolytes, especially if it's warm, at least twenty-four hours before your race starts.

Above half marathon distance

- If your race is on Saturday morning, ideally start thinking about carbohydrate intake on Tuesday, Wednesday and Thursday. On Friday, eat what feels most comfortable, but I usually suggest eating your main meal at lunchtime and having a lighter meal or snack in the evening to aid digestion. Don't forget to hydrate – using an electrolyte can help to ensure that you draw water into the body and muscles.

Contrary to what you may read, these carbohydrate-loading days are not about eating as much as you can – they are about trying to displace fat, fibre and some protein with carbohydrates. So your overall energy intake should not necessarily increase, but the percentage of carbohydrate intake should increase.

I personally find carbohydrate loading challenging. Not because I don't like carbohydrates – I love them – but as a small individual, I find the sheer volume of food difficult to manage. I have found using drinks helps to top up my carbohydrate intake from meals. My go-to is actually ginger beer, but you could use juice or a sports/carbohydrate drink mix and more easily digestible foods such as crumpets, hot cross buns, cake (usually carrot or banana for me) or even sweets.

One final thing to remember is that glycogen is stored in our muscles with water in a ratio of 1:3, so for every gram of glycogen, you will also hold 3 grams of water. This is also why you may feel quite full and heavy at a race start line. It is completely normal and the additional weight is not going to hinder your performance – quite the opposite.

Fuelling your training

Whether you are training for the track, 5k, 10k, marathon, ultra distance, road, trail, fells or mountains, chances are that your training week will consist of a mix of training sessions.

For those of you who are beginners, most of your runs will probably be done at an easy to steady state and last up to an hour. As your body starts to adapt and become stronger, you may find it beneficial to introduce shorter, faster sessions, especially if you are starting to think about targeting some races or running goals. However, I will always encourage you to work with a physio or qualified coach to ensure that you are not increasing volume, load or intensity too quickly.

For those of you who have been running for a few years and are at a stage where you are taking part in races regularly, a high percentage of your runs will probably be done at easy to steady state, but one to two runs per week are likely to include some intensity. This may be in the form of tempo running, intervals or hill reps. There will also be a longer run which will vary in distance depending on your specific goal.

Types of runs

1. High-intensity training session such as intervals, tempo or hills for up to sixty minutes

Ensuring sufficient fuelling in the twenty-four to thirty-six hours prior to these sessions is going to ensure that you have topped up your glycogen stores. However, when we are working at these very high work rates, our bodies can deplete our stores within forty-five minutes, so you may need to consider taking on fuel during the session to ensure that you can maintain the pace and intensity. This can also be beneficial if you know that your nutrition intake leading into the session hasn't been optimal due to work or life commitments. Having fuel on the go can mitigate this deficit to a degree.

I would recommend around 30–60 grams of carbohydrate an hour during one of these sessions. Aim to take on energy around twenty to thirty minutes into the session.

If you choose to fuel with gels, make sure that you take them on over a period of five minutes to allow for better absorption and ensure that you are hydrated. If you choose to fuel with a sports/carbohydrate mix drink, you will benefit from sipping on this throughout the session, maybe after each interval or hill, or in the minutes before and immediately after the tempo effort.

We will discuss alternatives to sports nutrition products a little later in this chapter.

2. Longer, moderate-intensity run of up to three hours

Once again, don't forget the importance of going into this session optimally fuelled.

During this type of training, you want to start thinking about fuelling twenty minutes into the run. These sessions are useful to practise race-day nutrition. Learning how your body responds to nutrition at higher paces, over different terrains and even in different conditions (such as rain, wind, snow and heat) is instrumental. Practising with your chosen fuel also ensures that you start to train your gut for race day. This is important for everyone, but especially if you are new to longer races or even races where you need to fuel.

The sports nutrition recommendations for these runs are 60–90 grams of carbohydrate per hour. To a certain degree, this will vary from individual to individual and even from run to run, especially in females.

The longer we are out on runs, fuelling is not the only thing we have to pay attention to and hydration is also key to maintain performance. Several studies confirm that as little as 2% dehydration can impact physical and cognitive performance significantly. Thus, the recommendations are to aim to consume 100–250 millilitres of fluid every twenty minutes, depending on conditions and the individual's losses. For example, fluid requirements increase at altitude or in hot climates (more on this shortly). Some individuals, myself included, may actually prefer to take on a lot of their energy through drinks, which means that you tackle fuelling, hydration and electrolytes all in one.

Finally, these runs are also a good opportunity to try caffeine. In general, gum releases caffeine into the body a lot faster than capsules or gels.

THE FEMALE FACTOR

In 2024 a study reported that out of articles published in six leading sports medicine and exercise journals from 2014 to 2020, only 6% exclusively studied women.[27] They concluded that this lack of research hinders the development of evidence-based, effective strategies to support the health, well-being and performance of female athletes to reach their full potential.

So although the recommendations for carbohydrate are 60–90 grams per hour, I have generally found in practice that a lot of women struggle to hit the top end, with the optimal being around 70 grams of carbohydrate per hour. However, if you are female and can tolerate more per hour without gastric distress, then this is still advised.

Similarly, although the lower end of carbohydrate intake during a run is set at 30 grams per hour, emerging studies are showing that the lowest threshold to support performance is actually 40 grams of carbohydrate per hour.

The other consideration for women is the potential hormonal influence over their requirements. Again, while studies are still quite scant, it has been shown that requirements for female runners increase during their luteal phase.[28]

While this will vary from individual to individual, it is also something I have observed in myself and in female athletes I work with.

When I am working with females who are not on hormonal contraception, I always encourage them to increase their intake of carbohydrate, both in their day-to-day nutrition and also in their long training runs and races, during the luteal phase of their cycle. Those who have taken on this advice have noticed improved performance at this stage of their cycle, improved energy levels generally and fewer fluctuations in mood.

Similarly, for active women who are in perimenopause or menopause, especially those who have chosen not to be on HRT, lower oestrogen levels actually mean that the body is more dependent on carbohydrate than it was prior to this phase of life.[29]

There is still so much we don't know about the female body and physiology. We have to make sensible decisions and approaches from the minimal but emerging studies that are available, but also use observational data, which I have plenty of from working with many female athletes and active individuals over the years.

While it is an exciting time for women's health, with so much attention and awareness being placed on it, it is also another opportunity for brands and organisations to profit from information and evidence that doesn't yet exist (more on this in chapter 8).

3. Longer trail runs over three hours

These runs will only really be necessary if you have signed up for an ultra-distance event. In general, whether you sign up for 50 miles or 100 miles, running the full distance ahead of race day is not recommended, as it places way too much stress on the body and takes a long time to recover from. This is also one of the reasons I worry so much about individuals who sign up for big events ranging from 50 kilometres up to 100 miles on a very regular basis, and don't leave enough time for their body to recover and repair. Personally, I only sign up to one or two races a year and ensure that they are pretty spread out so I get a chance to recover physically and psychologically.

As we have discussed in earlier chapters, while it can be difficult with so many individuals jumping on the running bandwagon and promoting race after race, it is really important to understand your running journey and choose races based on this (see the Reade and Bailey scale on page 23). This not only allows for longevity in running but also prolongs the enjoyment.

These runs are a perfect opportunity to test out fuelling strategies. It can be challenging to know how to fuel on ultraruns. From professional and personal experience, especially when you are running on trails, in the mountains or at altitude with constantly changing terrain and paces, there is room to include both sports nutrition and real food options.

A lot of the athletes I work with who run these longer distances find that they need to split their fuelling up. They might focus on solid fuel for the first part of the run, then maybe move more towards gels and jellies, finishing with liquid and caffeine. However, I cannot stress enough that you need to find the practice and options that work for you. I know some elites who can stomach gels even sixteen hours into races, while others can tuck into salted potatoes throughout 100 miles.

In these very long races, staying on top of hydration and sodium losses is critical; aiming for a minimum of 90 grams of carbohydrate per hour and trying to consume more without negative consequences is always going to result in a more consistent performance. While there is a move by some athletes to consume around 120 grams of carbohydrate per hour, it is important to appreciate that the studies associated with this trend are quite small, and that the most convincing was actually done on cyclists, not runners.

I have worked with a few elite runners recently where we have tried to push up the carbohydrate content per hour. This has had mixed results, and we have found that it often depends on the temperature. In hot climates, on the one hand, we need more carbohydrate as we utilise more in an attempt to keep our core temperature down; but at the same time, gastric emptying also slows down, which means that carbohydrate can sit in the digestive tract and lead to more gastric distress. It is a balancing act and the more you can practise, understand how your body responds and be open to adapting your strategy, the more successful this approach can be. From my observations, what seems to work best is general consistency in fuelling, rather than hitting an absolute number hourly. Thus during longer runs, especially those that also go through a night, we may find that we manage to consume higher amounts during the day, and then at night, due to our circadian rhythms (see chapter 7), we probably do better with a little less.

As runs and races get longer, there is now also guidance around taking on protein. In general, I recommend using a recovery drink at this stage – the combination of carbohydrates and protein makes it the perfect choice and also means that it is easily digestible. I highly recommend practising this in training because, once again, you may need to train your gut to tolerate this amount of protein on the go.

REAL FOOD FUEL

Here are some ideas that you may find useful to try as real food. You may have heard me saying on various podcasts that my go-tos are cheese and Marmite bagels, peanut brittle, Snickers and (as I've used at the Lakeland 50) my own version of a trail mix which includes Mini Cheddars, salted cashew nuts, peanut M&M's and sour sweets.

Some other options I've used with athletes across the years include:
- noodle soup
- oatcakes
- ginger cake
- Scotch pancakes
- pretzels
- wraps with a filling of choice, but good options include Marmite, peanut butter and banana, and cream cheese
- cereal bars
- salted peanuts
- salted potatoes
- flapjack
- Spanish omelette
- sushi (vegetarian)
- porridge pots
- pizza
- soya puddings
- flavoured milk
- pork pies

4. Fasted training

A few years ago, the term 'fasted training' was on everyone's lips, from recreational to elite athletes. While some endurance athletes still participate in this type of training, the majority are moving away from it.

Before we completely dismiss the idea, it is important to state that there is evidence to suggest that doing *some* training in a carbohydrate-depleted state may help you utilise more fat for fuel, which could be an advantage, particularly in endurance events where glycogen stores become depleted and are one of the limiting factors.

The theory is that if we help our body to adapt to utilising more fat as fuel, then we can spare our glycogen stores for longer. This concept is known as 'training low' and was first used in long-distance road cycling. However, as often is the case, scientific evidence gets misinterpreted, reworded and repackaged into something that is not strictly true, and yet becomes a way to generate financial gain for someone. Fasted training or training low is no exception to this rule: it has gone from training in a carbohydrate-depleted state to encouraging individuals to maintain low-carbohydrate intakes at all times as a way to lose more body fat and generally just be a bit confused and wary about carbohydrates.

What the science actually states is a little different. Training low does indeed involve training in a carbohydrate-depleted state, which is why many prefer to do this first thing and why it has become known as fasted training. BUT (and it's a big but) some key protocols need to be followed if an individual is to truly benefit.

- Firstly, these sessions should only be done *twice a week maximum.*
- Secondly, they should ideally only be *up to sixty minutes long and at an intensity that is no higher than a perceived exertion of six out of ten.*
- Finally, and most importantly, *you should still consume your overall carbohydrate requirements throughout the day.* If we think back to the theory from chapter 4, if your daily requirements are 5 grams of carbohydrate per kilogram of body weight, then you need to ensure that you do consume this, ideally evenly distributed throughout the rest of the day.

This final point is critical in order to actually get adaptation from training. Indeed, a meta-analysis of studies concluded that if individuals consumed low-carbohydrate intakes for three weeks or longer, there were negative implications for both health and performance in the long term.[30]

I do want to stress here that while this is a training approach you can include, it is absolutely not necessary. Studies have shown that endurance training, even with full glycogen stores, in itself also improves our ability to utilise more fat for fuel and is probably the preferred approach of most elite athletes and coaches.[31]

There are many reasons why I don't recommend fasted/depleted training. Firstly, the science is just not really stacked in favour of it. While there is some science to support the concept of training low, there are too many parameters, especially in understanding the exact pace or perceived exertion that actually allows for adaptation to happen. In my experience, very few people manage this well. Equally, many more studies discuss the negative implications of fasted training, both on performance and health.

Michael Gleeson, a professor at Loughborough University who I have had the pleasure of presenting alongside on several occasions at sports science conferences, has spoken for many years about the negative impact of low carbohydrate availability in athletes, especially associated with depressed immune systems.

As mentioned earlier, some runners choose to train fasted because they are under the misconception that it helps them to burn more fat and thus lose weight. This is not the case, and in fact the opposite is true. Fuelling your runs means you can work harder, provide the body with nutrients for cellular transcription and improve glycaemic control later in the day, thus supporting appetite control. In the few studies that have been done on women, it has been found that fasted training made no difference to body composition in comparison to fuelled training; indeed, the evidence suggests the opposite.

Fasted training can lead to a situation known as low energy availability, which in turn can underpin a condition called REDs, which I will go into much more detail about in chapter 8. Low energy availability is where there is not sufficient energy left over for biological health once the body has taken everything it needs for movement. The human body has evolved to prioritise energy for movement. Thus fasted training can create a situation for low energy availability to occur, especially if nutrition and particularly carbohydrate needs are not met throughout the rest of the day.

Although the odd day of low energy availability can be managed by the body, once it becomes prolonged (after a few weeks), it leads to a chronic rise in one of our stress hormones, cortisol. Similarly, training causes stress in the body. In addition, poor sleep or fewer hours of sleeping (under eight hours a night), being at a lower weight than your body naturally wants to be and the general stress of daily life all contribute to the overall stress in the body. When the stress associated with physical activity is prolonged or increased, it can also cause a rise in another stress hormone, prolactin. High levels of either or both of these stress hormones will be detected by the hypothalamus in the brain, resulting in a down-regulation of hormonal health. This in turn results in a decreased metabolism and turns on energy preservation and fat storage, poor adaptation from training, a depressed immune system, a decrease in bone cell production, and higher risk of injury and illness, to name a few consequences.

While this scenario can impact both men and women, we know that the female anatomy is more sensitive to it. Thus low energy availability, in particular low carbohydrate availability, has a real detrimental effect on both health and performance which may show up more quickly in women, but can similarly impact men.

When I'm working with runners, the most common reason stated for participating in fasted training is simply convenience. They like to train first thing before work, and the lack of available time can make it challenging to consume energy prior to training. However, it is clear that fuelling your morning training is not only advantageous for your health, but also for your performance and body composition. So how do you go about optimising your training with appropriate fuelling before an early morning session?

The most important thing to take on board is that we are not necessarily talking about eating a main breakfast. I definitely do not expect you to tuck into a hearty bowl of porridge and then get out of the door within twenty minutes. However, some good examples of easily digestible food options that can be consumed before a run include:

- a hot cross bun
- a glass of fruit juice and a banana
- a slice of toast with honey or jam
- 1 Weetabix with milk
- fruit yoghurt
- a sports gel – you could even have half before you leave the house and then the other half fifteen to twenty minutes into your run.

Post-run, aim to recover within thirty minutes with a good combination of carbohydrate and protein, to allow for optimal adaptation and progression, and a great start to the day.

5. Multi-day events

Multi-day events have become hugely popular. They can range upwards from two days where you might cover anything up to 100 kilometres over a weekend. They tend to be on trails, coastal paths or mountainous routes. They may be marked courses or require self-navigation to reach several checkpoints in a given time. Each day may have a specific cut-off. Some examples include Ultra X races, the Dragon's Back Race, the Great Lakeland 3Day, the OMM, the Jurassic Coast Challenge or my favourite, the Manaslu Trail Race in Nepal.

All of these events have overnight camps and may or may not provide food. There is a lot to think about with regard to your day-to-day nutrition and also in some cases your overnight nutrition. Most of these events have strict weight limits for your supporting bag, which is transported between camps while you run. For the Manaslu Trail Race, we had a 10-kilogram limit for all our kit, sleeping bag and trail food for eight stages. Thankfully, all our meals and a post-run recovery option were provided in ample quantites daily.

In contrast, there are races like the Spine Race and the Tor des Géants which are not technically stage races but have a certain number of days to complete the course and you decide when to stop and sleep. Both of these examples have aid stations where food and an option for sleeping are available.

I've personally done quite a few of these and my top tips are:

- As with previous runs, ensure that you start the event with full glycogen stores.
- Start fuelling within the first twenty to thirty minutes of your first day and continue every thirty to forty minutes, ideally aiming for your optimal amount per hour. I would advise practising in training and working out what is the highest amount you can consume.
- While a lot of these events involve more hiking and walking amongst the running, don't be fooled into thinking your requirements are not as high. Often the terrain or altitude will mean that you may be moving slower but you are definitely still utilising a lot of glucose per minute.
- Include protein sources during the day, especially in events where the days are long. In races like the Spine which are self-supported, you will have to carry these and ensure that you include them at regular intervals. It can be really useful to find a good recovery drink which you can make with water and which contains both carbohydrate and protein. At events like the Tor des Géants where you are allowed support and crew, you could ask them to provide flavoured milk at regular intervals to reduce the amount of muscle breakdown that will occur in these situations.
- Stay hydrated and on top of your salt losses (more on this shortly).

At the end of each running day, and this is probably more for events where there is a daily overnight camp, I would also suggest that you take on a recovery drink even before you start taking off your kit and getting warm or changing your socks. This is one of those scenarios where I think sports nutrition products really do have a role. Finding a recovery drink that you can just add water to, but which provides both carbohydrate and protein in an easily digestible form, really helps with optimising recovery between days. Obviously, you should also follow this up with a bit more of a substantial meal.

RUNNING AT ALTITUDE

Whether you are racing or training at altitude, there are some key considerations to take on board. Generally speaking, we start to feel the effects of altitude above 2,000 metres, although this varies from person to person. When we are at altitude, our respiratory rate increases, which means that our fluid requirements are much higher. Dehydration is one of the most common causes for nausea at altitude and staying on top of fluid intake is critical. Similarly, as our bodies are working harder, the advice is to go slower but also increase our carbohydrate intake, both during the activity and around it at mealtimes. Personally, I find that my appetite increases when I am at altitude, but some people find that they lose their appetite, especially over 3,000 metres where a cough known as 'altitude cough' can occur. In these situations, it is important to eat mechanically regardless of appetite.

Fuelling on runs can be quite challenging. In 2023 I returned to my beloved Nepal, this time to do the Mustang Trail Race. We were heading over 4,000-metre passes daily. All of us found it very challenging hiking up to high altitudes, especially with poles, while also trying to eat and swallow food. I used more liquid energy in the form of carbohydrate mixes, but one tip I highly recommend is sucking on boiled sweets. I took a mix of options, from mints to lemon sherbets and orange barleys. This helped to prevent my mouth from getting too dry, and also ensured that a small amount of glucose was constantly reaching my brain. While it wasn't enough to meet my hourly requirements for carbs, this process of 'carbohydrate rinsing' tricked my brain into thinking energy was available, which meant that I could maintain my pace, albeit not very fast!

Similarly, my friend and editor Kirsty recently did the Tor des Géants. After her first night, she sent me a voice note saying she was feeling really nauseous and struggling to eat anything. I am familiar with the route and knew she had done some big climbs through the night. We often forget the effect of altitude and think we can continue to work at the same rate as on a hill back home. I advised her to slow down on the climbs just a little, drink more, suck boiled sweets and wait it out. After three days, she sent me another voice note to say she was feeling so much better and had just managed to eat an amazing focaccia sandwich which was the best sandwich she had ever eaten.

I have one final point to make, which refers more to training at altitude: a lot of runners go out to altitude to improve their production of red blood cells and thus hopefully improve performance back at sea level. Be mindful that if you are in low energy availability and your iron stores are low (less than 50 micrograms per litre), you will not get any training benefits at altitude. Therefore, it is worth ensuring that your values are good before you head out to the mountains.

6. Rest days

While these are not technically a type of run, I do feel that they are equally as important to include. As I've pointed out earlier, a rest day is an opportunity for your body to catch up, take stock, recover and adapt.

However, in the crazy world we live in, with all the noise, especially in the arena of running and fitness, taking a rest day can almost seem like a sign of weakness. Interestingly, among the runners I work with, most of the elite and professional runners take rest days, while everyday runners often choose not to and then wonder why they are not progressing and why they get injured.

There is no set day to have a rest day. Personally, I vary this – some weeks I have one; other weeks and months I opt to have two or more. When I first started running, I actually ran three times a week and didn't do any additional activity on the other days apart from walking and pushing the buggy around.

A lot of the elites I work with follow more of a 'ten days on, one day off' system. As I say, it is all very personal, but a regular full day of rest is highly recommended, and no, you don't have to eat less on these days, even if it is more than once a week. Please remember that the body is generally in a constant state of flux and is not absolute, so it is always monitoring and working out how to maintain balance.

I am a great believer in listening to your own body and responding – if it is tired, why push it? What is this actually going to achieve? And stop comparing yourself to those around you. We are all different, all experiencing our own bodies, and all have to find the approach that is appropriate and relevant to us at that moment.

Eating on the move

In the previous section, we spoke a lot about the importance of fuelling our runs, but I know this is not something that everyone finds easy to do. One of the most common issues runners speak to me about is the experience of gastric distress during runs and races, which then prevents them from fuelling.

It is evident how important carbohydrate availability is, not just for our running performance but also for our overall health and ability to repair, recover and adapt from training. However, from my observations and assessments working with runners, it is clear that many of them avoid fuelling during training. Although they still understand the importance of fuelling when it comes to race day, their body has not learnt how to tolerate fuel on the go. When I ask them why this is the case, the majority respond with the notion that they prefer to 'save' their energy for after training, so they have something to look forward to.

This is definitely one myth I want to rectify. I've said it previously, but providing your body with sufficient energy – especially carbohydrates, before, during and after your runs – not only supports optimal performance and recovery, but also helps with satiety and managing appetite.

Everyone will have their own personal preference when it comes to race-day nutrition. This will also depend on the type of race – supported or unsupported, at altitude or in the desert, hot or cold, road or trails, single-day or multi-day, and how long each day will be.

Ideally, especially if you are using sports nutrition products, fuel needs to be in the form of glucose and fructose, both of which are simple sugars but with slightly different molecular structures. For some context, the body is able to absorb around 60 grams of glucose and 30 grams of fructose per hour, so in a 2:1 ratio. Some studies are emerging that suggest that this upper limit of 90 grams in total could be increased to 120 grams in some athletes who train their guts. Interestingly, the ratio of glucose to fructose has been altered as it has been found that glucose absorption tops out at 60 grams per hour, but there appears to be some room for manoeuvre with fructose, which can be added to increase overall intake. That said, at present, no ideal or optimal ratio has been determined. I have worked with a few elite athletes recently where we have tried ratios of 1:1 and also 0.8:1. To date, the 1:1 ratio was better tolerated in running, but even then it was not something that could be taken on continuously and intake did need to alter through the course of the run. We definitely need more research in this area, but for now what I will say is that whatever you choose, the key is practise, practise, practise until you have nailed what works for you, and don't be scared to vary it.

Here are some of the most common mistakes I have observed in runners, especially those that lead to gastric distress:

- Leaving it too long before starting fuelling; ideally, you want to start taking on nutrition within the first thirty minutes and continue every thirty to forty minutes.
- Taking sports gels too quickly; aim to take one gel over four or five minutes rather than all in one go. This helps with absorption and tolerance.
- Becoming dehydrated and not taking on replacing fluids and electrolytes, specifically sodium.
- Trying new products on race day.

Hydration and electrolytes

Hydration is something a lot of people neglect, when in reality it is crucial to your running and race success. It is well documented in scientific literature that fluid intake and adequate hydration are essential during exercise, and critical during prolonged training sessions and endurance races.

The key role of fluid intake during endurance running is to maintain hydration, thermoregulation (body temperature) and adequate plasma (blood) volume, and to avoid dehydration.

Ensuring that plasma volume and thermoregulation stay within an optimal range has a direct impact on performance. When core body temperature rises due to dehydration, plasma volume decreases, resulting in an increased heart rate, which accelerates fatigue. Just a 1% reduction in body weight through fluid losses can contribute to these negative physiological effects. In addition, dehydration has a marked effect on cognitive function, resulting in an inability to make decisions.

And what about salts? Most runners will sweat between 400 and 2,400 millilitres per hour of exercise, with the average value being around 1,200 millilitres per hour, although this will vary with age, sex, weight, the intensity of running and the environmental temperature. These sweat losses are predominantly water, but the main electrolyte lost is sodium.

The sodium content of sweat varies substantially, from 115 milligrams to more than 2,000 milligrams per 1,000 millilitres of sweat. A runner who is a 'salty sweater' (that is, who has a high amount of sodium in their sweat) may lose well in excess of the recommended intakes. While sodium losses can impact any race, they are more likely to be problematic in longer endurance races, particularly marathon distance and upwards.

Salt losses are very individual, but as a rule of thumb I suggest that runners need to take around 700–900 milligrams of sodium per litre of fluid, particularly during ultra-distance events. This point around the amount per litre is critical, and is the reason why so many people get into trouble. During races where you are usually constantly refilling soft flasks and topping up water intakes, it can be easy to lose sight of how much fluid you have had and how much sodium you have diluted within the volume you have consumed.

Sodium can be consumed in a number of ways – salt tablets, electrolytes, energy drinks and even food. Some good food suggestions include salted peanuts, mashed potato with cheese or Marmite, cheese straws and cured meat.

It is important to appreciate that most electrolyte tablets, salt capsules or sports drinks will only provide around 250–300 milligrams of sodium. Personally, I have found a combination of chewable electrolytes, sodium in my carb mix and real food to be a pretty good way to meet my requirements. For the record, I have very high sodium losses. While I've never done sweat tests, which are quite popular and useful to a degree, I know I have high losses because there are always large white patches from salt crystals on my T-shirt and running pack, and I can also taste the salt in my sweat.

Back in 2019 I signed up for and started the Ultra Tour Monte Rosa stage race, which covers 170 kilometres in four days. On day one, I had just reached the final aid station for the day and another runner was having a really tough time with nausea. He was chatting to the medics and they didn't appear to understand what might be wrong with him. Technically I was off duty, but I always find it hard not to help if I can, so I asked him what was going on. He explained that he was feeling really sick and couldn't keep food or liquid down. It had been a pretty warm day. I asked him how much fluid and salt he had taken on. He said lots of fluid but no salt. He had packed salt capsules but hadn't bothered to bring them out on the first day as he didn't think it was going to be warm enough. I gave him some of my salt capsules and told him to take a few, which would help to draw some water into his body, and then to just sit it out for a bit and start running once he felt less nauseous.

I left him at this stage – it was a race, after all, and what was left was a beautiful descent into Zermatt. After I had a quick wash and took on some recovery, I headed back to the finish line to watch others complete the first day. As I approached the finish line, the same guy had just crossed it. He saw me and just said he was so grateful. His nausea had passed and he had really enjoyed the second half of the day.

On the second day, we set off in the early hours of the morning on a huge climb to a glacier. There was then another really big climb through a forest and up to the refuge. I was really struggling. The temperature had risen once again and it was actually quite humid.

I made it to the refuge but felt rubbish with nausea. I ate some bread and cheese, filled my bottles and thought, *I just have to get this day done.* As I ran down from the refuge, I remember that familiar sloshing in the stomach which I knew was lack of salt. I was so thirsty but just hadn't taken enough sodium on because I had made a rookie error: after giving some of my salt tablets away the previous day, I had forgotten to repack any. I had hoped that my carb mix would be sufficient, but sadly it was not.

I remember getting to a point where I felt a bit beaten. I sat on a rock and just hoped someone would pass by and have some spare salt tablets. As it happened, within twenty minutes, the guy I had helped out the day before stopped and asked if I was okay. I explained my situation. He said he had loads of salt tablets on him and I could have as many as I wanted. I took two and felt better within fifteen to twenty minutes. Karma!

We ran the rest of that day together and made it back just before the weather changed again, this time to heavy rain which sadly stopped the race for everyone that year. It's still a race I want to go back and finish at some point.

SYMPTOMS OF LOW SODIUM

Low sodium intakes and dehydration are very common in runners, especially those of us who participate in ultrarunning. Remember that sodium helps to draw water into your body and the working muscles. If you are someone who has high sodium losses and you don't replace them appropriately, even if you keep drinking, your body will not be able to absorb this fluid and thus it can often feel like a washing machine in your stomach.

Female runners also need to be aware that our sodium losses change across the menstrual cycle. Once again during the luteal phase, post-ovulation, when progesterone is dominant, we have higher sweat rates in an attempt to keep our core temperature down, and thus have higher sodium losses. So, like carbohydrate, you may have to adjust your sodium strategy for race day if it falls at this point in your cycle.

So, what are the symptoms often associated with hyponatremia or low sodium?

- Gastrointestinal distress
- Nausea
- Bloating
- Fatigue
- Impaired concentration
- Dizziness
- Heat stress

One of the most common causes of stomach issues during runs and races is related to sodium and fluid balance, not the sports nutrition gel or bar that most runners allude to.

Comparatively, it is important to highlight that it can be just as easy to overconsume sodium and this too can cause stomach issues. A key sign is if you notice you are urinating more frequently, more often than every twenty minutes, or have very frequent bouts of diarrhoea, which could actually suggest hypernatremia (too much sodium). In this case, it's a good idea to back off the salt tablets for a short time, take on fluid and let the body reset and then start taking electrolytes back on, potentially at a lower dose.

Sodium and fluid balance is a definite juggling act and you need to learn to adapt, especially during long ultra-distance races. Understanding some of these symptoms and learning to adjust on the go will definitely put you in good stead.

Finally, sodium balance and staying hydrated is not just confined to during running; it is equally important to think about leading into an event. I regularly recommend that individuals start drinking electrolytes, in a value tailored to their event, in the twenty-four hours prior to the start of their race.

CHAPTER 7

Top tips and example menus

Top tips

Before I move on to choices of sports nutrition products, I wanted to share some of my top tips with you. These are little nuggets of gold I've learnt through hands-on experience over the course of my career. They include pieces of information I've gained through my own learning and research when supporting elite runners, and also some personal lessons.

Contingency planning

One of the most important learning outcomes from my time working with the GB wheelchair basketball and wheelchair fencing teams going into Rio 2016 was always having a plan but always having a contingency plan too. This probably relates to all racing, but particularly to long distances or racing over multiple days.

It is very unlikely that you will ever cover the full distance of your chosen event in training, especially if it is longer than the marathon distance. It can be easy to assume that your chosen fuel is going to work hour after hour, day after day. However, I have definitely become unstuck with this and I know from talking to many of my friends and the runners I work with that this is a common mistake.

This is why when I became team manager for the GB 24-hour team, I would ask the runners for their fuelling strategy weeks ahead of the championships and then ensure that they also had a Plan B and Plan C. This process gives you confidence, so that when there is inevitably a problem, you don't panic and you know that there is something else you can try.

Learn to adapt

Even with all the planning and practising before an event, there are always races where things don't pan out how you expect. Maybe the weather throws you or you have a kit failure or you are just not feeling it that day. Learning to be adaptive in the moment is a key skill that is often the difference between runners who finish races and those who don't.

For example, if the weather conditions are atrocious, the likelihood of getting a personal best or even an expected time goal is small. However, if you can accept this and move your goal, it can often help you manage your mindset in a race.

It is also important to hold on to the fact that, for the majority of us who run for enjoyment and participation, it is just running. It is not something to hold your wrath against, and definitely not something that should cause psychological distress.

CASE STUDY

In summer 2024, my friend Shane Ohly, CEO of Ourea Events and race director of the Dragon's Back Race (DBR), decided to attempt an FKT (fastest known time) for the whole distance of the DBR in one go. He was meticulous in his planning and training. He practised his race nutrition and we had a few discussions in the lead-up to his attempt. He was amazing and completed the 380 kilometres from Conwy to Cardiff Castle in 102 hours and 33 minutes.

When I caught up with Shane after the attempt, he told me that food had been one of the hardest components to get right. Even though he had had all the best intentions and so many food options, after a couple of days he started to get such a sore mouth that he really struggled to eat. A lot of runners who do these very long attempts describe this, and it is usually a side effect of the stress the body has been placed under. Some top tips include using antibacterial mouthwash regularly and having some soft foods like porridge pots, soya puddings and noodles in soup.

Nausea

Nausea is a common problem, and we are inevitably going to notice it at some point during a long endurance effort. As we've discussed previously, sodium and fluid balance often contribute to this, but effort and terrain, especially altitude, can also have a part to play. Nausea is also a side effect from fatigue. To a certain degree, it is a consequence of having chosen to put your body in such an extreme place.

However, there are things that can help. Ginger is a big one, and crystalline chews, ginger beer or sports nutrition that is made from ginger can be game-changers. Sucking a boiled sweet is another trick to have up your sleeve.

The key thing is to not stop eating. No matter how little the quantity, keep putting small amounts into your body at regular intervals. Once you stop fuelling, it impacts not only your physical performance but also your mindset.

Circadian rhythm

Circadian rhythm is attributed to the twenty-four-hour internal clock in our brain that regulates cycles of alertness and sleepiness by responding to light changes in our environment. This biological circadian system has evolved to help us adapt to changes in our environment and anticipate changes in radiation, temperature and food availability.[32] New research is emerging looking at the impact our circadian rhythm has on nutritional intakes, especially in races that go through the night.

In normal circumstances, the body is often preparing for sleep at night and alongside this come adjustments in digestion. For runners doing races that start at night or go through the night, it is easier on the gut and more advantageous to performance to make some adjustments to intake, especially reducing the carbohydrate per hour to slightly less than that consumed during the day. There is also some evidence that eating more protein-based foods can keep you more alert at night. So, while I would definitely not displace all the carbohydrates with protein, adding some cheese, nuts, soya puddings or cartons of flavoured milk into the mix may support performance.

Do we really need sports nutrition products?

Sports nutrition was formulated in response to advances in sport science. As we became more and more aware of how our bodies utilise fuel during exercise and what the limiting factors are, sports brands started considering how they could support individuals participating in training and performance, but also how they could diversify their income.

One case in point is Lucozade. Remember the golden-coloured liquid that was equally promoted as an energy drink in sport and as an aid to support individuals who had experienced illness and lost their appetite as a result? Years later, they introduced a sport-specific drink. It still boasted the benefits of providing energy for those participating in sport, but had added electrolytes and was branded as isotonic, which encourages absorption and rehydration, and it was available in vending machines in sports centres up and down the country.

Over the years, sports nutrition has continued to evolve, moving from drinks to gels to chews to bars, playing around in composition and always trying to provide that extra edge to our performance. With ultra-distance sports taking centre stage a lot more, product formulations have altered to be specific for these needs. However, while there is ample choice, the cost of all this nutrition can sometimes be difficult to swallow, especially based on the amounts and volumes often suggested by the brands.

As a professional working in sports nutrition and also someone who runs, I get to test and try products that are sent to me by many sports nutrition brands. I rarely put my name to something unless my values align with the brand, and I often wrestle with recommending a product, especially when there is a price tag attached to it.

That said, in certain situations, sports nutrition does have its place in creating and delivering an ideal mix of nutrients, hydration and electrolytes to active bodies. For example, in road races, 10-kilometre races, half marathons or marathons, due to the faster pace, runners are generally likely to benefit from taking on fuel that is easily digestible. In my case, I can't even chew food at this pace, so the only types of fuel I could possibly take are gels or carbohydrate mixes.

Similarly, as we discussed earlier, in ultra-distance events, electrolytes or carbohydrate mixes that have been formulated with a higher sodium content are useful and important to those runners who have very high sodium losses and for whom food alone is not going to be sufficient. That said, if you were basing all your requirements on sports nutrition alone, you might find the sheer volume not only a lot to finance but also quite heavy to carry. Your body might also get to a point where by hour twelve it could no longer stomach a raspberry-cheesecake-flavoured gel which tasted great at hour one.

Another scenario where sports nutrition takes precedence over real food is in races abroad, multi-day events or long distances over 100 kilometres, where you will benefit from including a recovery drink which has both carbohydrates and protein and can be made up with water alone.

Equally, there are situations, means and ways in which you can still meet your requirements without paying the price.

STRAIGHT SWAPS

The average gel usually has in the region of 20–30 grams of carbohydrate, depending on the brand. Similarly, sports chews have also become very popular, with the average serving (three or four chews) providing around 30–40 grams of carbohydrate.

The equivalent would be:
- a medium-sized banana (not the easiest to transport, but useful for training runs)
- five or six regular-sized jelly babies
- two 16-gram packets of Haribo Starmix
- two small boxes of raisins
- four pitted dates.

However, before you become overzealous with the dried fruit, remember that overconsuming fructose can contribute to higher rates of gastrointestinal distress, especially during runs.

Ready-prepared sports drinks, such as Lucozade and Gatorade, provide 30 grams of carbohydrate per 500 millilitres and 20–30 millimoles of sodium. A simple alternative is to dilute 300 millilitres of orange juice with 300 millilitres of water and add a quarter of a teaspoon of salt, which gives you exactly the same composition.

One area where you rarely need to use a specific targeted sports-nutrition product is in recovery. Studies have repeatedly demonstrated that cow's milk or flavoured cow's milk is an excellent recovery choice. In fact, most of the recovery drink options on the market are based on milk and its nutritional profile, as it provides the exact mix of carbohydrate, protein, electrolytes and hydration needed for optimal recovery.

However, it is important to point out that some of the plant-based drinks are not quite as nutrient-dense, so don't always deliver. Those of you who are plant-based may have to be mindful of this. For example, having a carton of chocolate soya milk with a banana will ensure that any discrepancies in nutrition are met.

TOP TIPS

- Good options for pre-fuel include flapjacks, banana bread or a fruit-juice-based smoothie.
- Good options for recovery include flavoured milk or recovery smoothies – try blending frozen fruit, milk and Greek-style yoghurt with a squeeze of honey for a quick and easy recipe.
- For colder days, how about a recovery hot chocolate? Try using milk fortified with skimmed milk powder to enhance the protein content.

Recovery goals

So, we have discussed nutrition for fuelling and nutrition during your runs, but what about after your run?

After each run, training session or race, runners need to be mindful about their recovery, ensuring that ideally they take this on within thirty minutes of finishing. The recommendations are 1.2 grams of carbohydrate per kilogram of body weight, and up to 0.4 grams of protein per kilogram of body weight. If this is not a timed meal, then a recovery snack needs to be consumed, which could be something like:

- a recovery drink with both carbohydrate and protein
- a carton of flavoured milk with a cereal bar or banana
- Greek yoghurt with granola
- a recovery smoothie as mentioned in the last box.

Just as a caveat, these are examples but intakes will have to vary depending on your requirements using the equation above.

These recovery options ensure a good intake of carbohydrate and protein to start the replenishment process. This should then be followed up with a balanced meal within two hours. The recovery option is particularly important when there are fewer than twelve hours until your next training session, regardless of whether this is a strength session later in the day or another run, perhaps the morning after an evening run.

I have already discussed the negative implications of fasted runs. One key issue is when runners insist on doing a run depleted and their run is also at a high intensity. As we heard earlier, the resulting increase in stress hormones can be problematic. However, it is also common for appetite to be reduced after such hard sessions. This is because when we train hard, blood flow is directed away from our stomach and towards our working muscles. There is usually a lag period while blood flow returns to normal, and this is the key reason why so many of us struggle to feel hungry after training. While delaying your recovery snack may seem immaterial, it can contribute to poor recovery between run sessions and also low energy availability.

Ghrelin is our hunger hormone. Levels rise after exercise or several hours after a meal, signifying that we need to refuel. Leptin is a hormone that helps regulate appetite, energy balance and other physiological processes, including menstrual health in females. Leptin is released from adipose tissue (body fat) and helps maintain a normal weight by making us feel full.

When ghrelin is high, leptin levels are low. Both these hormones return to normal levels when energy demands are met. However, if a runner continually fails to fuel adequately after a training session, intentionally or unintentionally, leptin levels stay low. Chronic low leptin levels send a signal to the body to encourage energy preservation. So, while the runner may think they are going to lose weight and improve body composition, the reverse can happen. It's important to highlight here that this is a simplified version to help explain why some runners, even when they restrict intake or increase training, still don't achieve the body composition and weight goals they would expect.

Example day menus

Now we have all the information, how does this actually translate into practice?

In order to provide you with some guidance, I have shared a few example day menus. I want to stress that they are just examples to help you make informed and appropriate decisions, especially around nutrient timing and composition. Amounts and choices of actual macronutrients can all be altered to meet your personal preference.

Example 1: early morning easy run

You should never do fasted training as this will depress the immune system and increase your levels of the stress hormone cortisol, which affects your metabolism and body composition.

Early morning: if you struggle to eat, some good options are:
- a slice of toast with jam or honey
- a glass of juice and a banana
- a fruit yoghurt
- a hot cross bun
- 1 Weetabix with milk
- sports gel or chews.

Recover within thirty minutes of completing your run. If this can't be your next meal, then take on 300 millilitres of cow's milk and whey shake, followed by your next meal.

Breakfast options include:
- two or three boiled, scrambled or poached eggs on two slices of wholegrain toast or a toasted wholegrain bagel. Add mushrooms and tomatoes for added nutrients
- 150 grams of Greek yoghurt with a large serving of muesli and fruit
- Bircher muesli (this can be made the night before)
- a wholegrain bagel with nut butter and a banana with a glass of juice
- two pieces of toast with half a tin of baked beans and a glass of juice
- a large serving of porridge made with milk and topped with toasted walnuts and honey.

Lunch: a portion of carbs, a portion of protein, a portion of essential fats and salad or vegetables, followed by Greek yoghurt and fruit. Some examples include:
- one or two large wholemeal pittas with hummus and a vibrant salad with tomatoes, cucumber, leaves, avocado, grated carrots and beetroot, served with balsamic vinegar or lemon/lime juice
- a serving of vegetable and bean hot pot with a large jacket or baked sweet potato
- a medium jacket potato with a small tin of baked beans and salad

- a salmon wrap
- roasted veg bruschetta
- a bowl of home-made soup and a cheese toastie
- a tuna melt. Slice one wholemeal ciabatta or sourdough roll in half and spread a small can of tuna evenly between both halves. Top with grated cheese and place under a medium grill for a few minutes until the cheese has melted. Top with sliced cucumber and serve immediately.

Mid-afternoon snack choice:
- malt loaf and a 300-millilitre glass of milk
- a fruit smoothie
- toast with avocado and feta or peanut butter and banana
- a bowl of cereal with fruit
- crumpets with fruit and 100 grams of Greek yoghurt
- three or four oatcakes with mackerel pâté, cream cheese or hummus.

Evening meal: a portion of carbs, a portion of protein, veg or salad; and yoghurt, honey and fruit. Examples include:
- vegetable and cheese frittata served with two slices of wholegrain toast or a jacket potato
- chicken or tofu stir fry
- a large jacket potato with tuna mayonnaise and salad
- vegetable red Thai curry served with rice
- fish pie served with vegetables
- sausage casserole with couscous or baked potato.

Example 2: rest day
Breakfast: choose one of the following:
- two or three boiled, scrambled or poached eggs on two slices of wholegrain toast or a toasted wholegrain bagel
- 150 grams of yoghurt with 60 grams of muesli and fruit
- Bircher muesli
- a wholegrain bagel with nut butter and a banana with a glass of juice
- two pieces of toast with half an avocado mashed and a glass of juice
- porridge made with milk, topped with toasted walnuts and honey.

Lunch:
- a third of a plate of nutrient-dense wholegrain carbohydrate
- a third of a plate of (smartphone-sized) protein
- a third of a plate of vegetables/salad – aim for a variety of colours to maximise antioxidants
- a thumb-sized portion of essential fats
- follow with Greek yoghurt, fruit and honey.

Mid-afternoon snack choice:
- a matchbox-sized portion of cheese and apple
- a latte
- two boiled eggs
- 30 grams of nuts
- avocado and feta dip (half an avocado plus 30 grams of feta) with carrots
- mackerel pâté (one fillet of smoked mackerel with 20 grams of cream cheese and lemon juice) with veg.

Evening meal:
- a third of a plate of nutrient-dense wholegrain carbohydrate
- a third of a plate of (smartphone-sized) protein
- a third of a plate of vegetables/salad – aim for a variety of colours to maximise antioxidants
- a thumb-sized portion of essential fats
- follow with Greek yoghurt, fruit and honey.

Before bed:
- a milk-based drink such as hot chocolate – try melting two squares of good quality chocolate into 300 millilitres of milk.

Example 3: long run or higher-intensity run session

Breakfast: carb-based, such as:
- a toasted bagel with peanut butter and banana
- pancakes with Greek yoghurt and berries
- porridge with honey and banana.

Fuel your run as recommended in chapter 6 (pages 102–114) depending on duration and intensity.

Post-run: recover immediately with a recovery shake made with cow's or oat milk and then a main meal as soon as possible:
- a third of a plate of nutrient-dense wholegrain carbohydrate
- a third of a plate of (smartphone-sized) protein
- a third of a plate of vegetables/salad – aim for a variety of colours to maximise antioxidants
- a thumb-sized portion of essential fats.

Mid-afternoon snack choice:
- cereal bar or flapjack or piece of cake with a milk-based drink
- oatcakes or equivalent with peanut butter and banana
- Greek yoghurt with fruit, oats, muesli or granola – sweeten with honey as needed
- dried fruit and nuts
- half an avocado (with feta) mashed on toast
- two slices of fruit bread or similar with butter.

Evening meal:
- a third of a plate of nutrient-dense wholegrain carbohydrate
- a third of a plate of (smartphone-sized) protein
- a third of a plate of vegetables/salad – aim for a variety of colours to maximise antioxidants
- a thumb-sized portion of essential fats
- follow with Greek yoghurt, fruit and honey.

Later in the evening: a glass of milk with a snack such as:
- two oatcakes with a topping of choice
- a piece of toast with a topping of choice
- a small bowl of cereal.

Final word on fuelling for training

Fuelling for training is critical if you want to get optimal adaptation and progression. Understanding what you need to consume before, during and after training is fundamental to performance. Intra-run fuelling is going to be necessary in certain training situations. You also need to consider the terrain, distance and time on your feet, as these all have implications to energy requirements.

Everyone will have their own personal preferences when it comes to nutrition, and specifically race-day nutrition. This will also depend on the type and length of race. For example, those running on trails or mixed terrain often prefer to use real food during training and races. This works as there will be fluctuations in pace, which means that food may be better tolerated in comparison to someone doing a flat-out road run where all blood flow has been directed away from the stomach and into the working muscles, making it more difficult to digest solid food.

In all situations, it is important to practise with your race-day choices through training to allow the gut to adapt. On that note, remember that fruit and dried fruit has a high fructose content, so be mindful of how much you consume as this can potentially cause digestive issues during your race or training.

Another key piece to the puzzle is monitoring. In order to understand how you are responding and adapting to training, keep a close eye on recovery, immunity, hormonal and stress biomarkers to ensure that you can adjust nutritional strategies accordingly. When I am working with elite athletes, I do this fairly regularly, usually after high training volume blocks or big races.

For most of us who are everyday runners, I would definitely recommend a once-a-year MOT as a minimum to check markers such as vitamin D, ferritin, thyroid function, creatine phosphokinase, cortisol and reproductive hormones. Contact your GP in the first instance.

In addition, it is imperative to do a daily monitoring score around readiness to train, fatigue scores and how a training session feels, in order to ensure that training load is managed appropriately and adequate rest is scheduled in.

Finally, make it individual – take on board the fundamental practices and then work out what you like. There is nothing worse than trying to consume something you can't stand the taste of just because it has been written somewhere that it is good for you, or your training buddy swears by it. If you don't like the taste of something, you are unlikely to consume it, especially under race-day conditions when pressure can be high. The key objective is to work out what is practical and easy to source, and to know that you can tolerate it.

PART 3

Humans are not textbooks

CHAPTER 8

False refuges and how they hinder us

Those of you who know me and follow my work will know that one of the things I deplore the most is disingenuity. I will call out misinformation and make it my mission not only to educate but to advocate for those who are vulnerable.

So this chapter will look at some of the situations that can derail your relationship with running and hinder your performance. I will discuss mistakes I see all the time, provide you with a comprehensive guide of dos and don'ts, and create a list for medics and other allied health professionals who may not be aware of some of the differences between the general population and runners.

I think it is fair to say that no one's relationship with running is linear. Work, family, illness or injury will come along and potentially derail it at some point. While these are likely to be minor setbacks, at times they can be major.

With my own running journey, I've only really had one major injury if we don't include my sarcoidosis diagnosis, and it came because I chose not to listen to my body and got caught up in external noise. Lesson learnt, though, and since that point I've been super mindful of what information I absorb and also very diligent about choosing training that is appropriate and relevant to me and my body, including strength/resistance training.

Indeed, external noise is one of the key problems with the society we live in now, with so many of us sharing intricate details of our lives. Professional athletes, run-fluencers, the general population, we all want to create highlight reels showcasing who we are. Our identities have become entangled in our online presence, and many of us are actually failing to look inwardly and ask: 'What is going on for me? What do I need right now?' And of course, if we choose to follow one type of identity, that will then be what informs us, creates thoughts and beliefs, and ultimately impacts our behaviours.

I often speak about the perfect storm that combines our personality type with psychosocial factors that impact our internal dialogue and thus our behaviours.

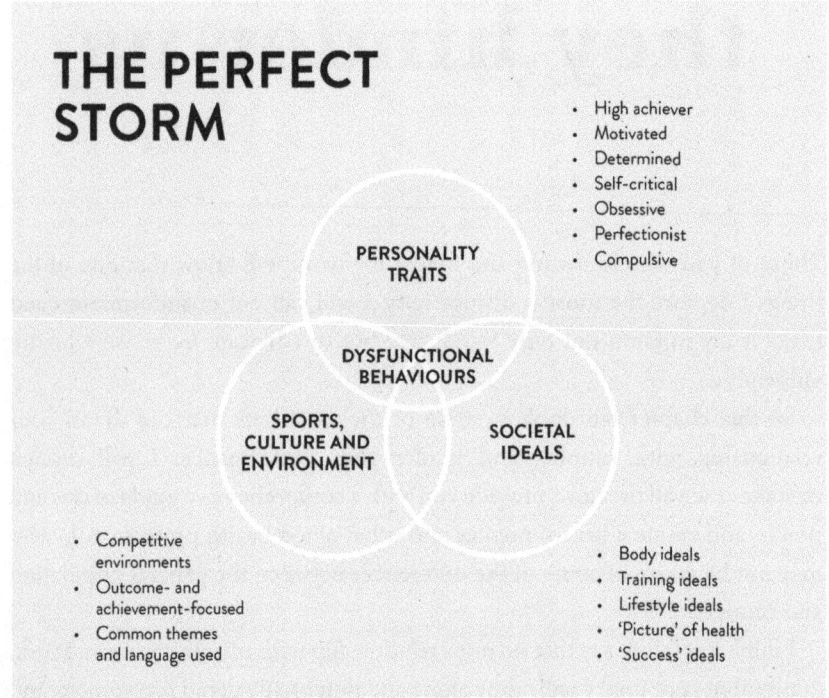

Figure 8.1

What we can see from figure 8.1 is that particular types of personality are often more susceptible to dysfunctional behaviours, small or large. You put these traits into specific environments and then add societal messaging and pressures and you create the perfect storm for dysfunctional behaviours to develop. These may feel like the right approach in that moment, often because they alleviate an underlying sense of 'There is something wrong with me', 'I'm not okay' or 'I'm falling short.' Sadly, these behaviours act as a bit of a sticking plaster. They hold back these difficult emotions temporarily but the relief is short-lived.

Limiting beliefs and dysfunctional behaviours

You may be wondering why I have called this chapter 'False refuges'. I am going to be honest, it is not a term I have coined but it is one I borrow a lot from Tara Brach when I am trying to explain certain behaviours to those I work with.

In the opening chapters of this book, I spoke candidly about my concern regarding the rise of run-fluencers and the content they put out. Many of them create unrealistic ideals and expectations that, albeit not intentionally, set many people up to fail. The noise they create can lead us to develop limiting beliefs about ourselves, which in turn lead to dysfunctional behaviours. It is these dysfunctional behaviours that I call false refuges, because they provide a false sense of security.

Limiting beliefs are beliefs that keep us stuck in a place that is not productive or purposeful. For example, you might believe that being lighter will make you faster but ignore the fact that by dropping weight you actually hold your body at a place that is not optimal for you. In this example, it is also important to point out when someone does initially lose weight or make a change to their body composition, they may indeed get one or two great performances, which helps to cement the validity of this belief. However, there is often a lag period where the body is adjusting but also trying to maintain equilibrium. This is why you get a couple of good performances and then the body can no longer sustain performance because the foundations of biological health have become compromised. The belief is so strong that even with deteriorating performance and increased occurrence of niggles and injuries, you maintain behaviours that keep your body at a place where it can't function for you. This belief limits your potential, but the emotions around it are so strong that you are too afraid to restore weight and see how it may impact (and probably improve) your health and performance.

While I don't believe that run-fluencers directly cause this type of thinking, their content contributes to noise and soundbites that many of us ingest and, instead of filtering, turn into facts and beliefs, leading to dysfunctional behaviours or false refuges. This is especially true when run-fluencers share training sessions, post 'what I eat in a day' videos or discuss the supplements they take.

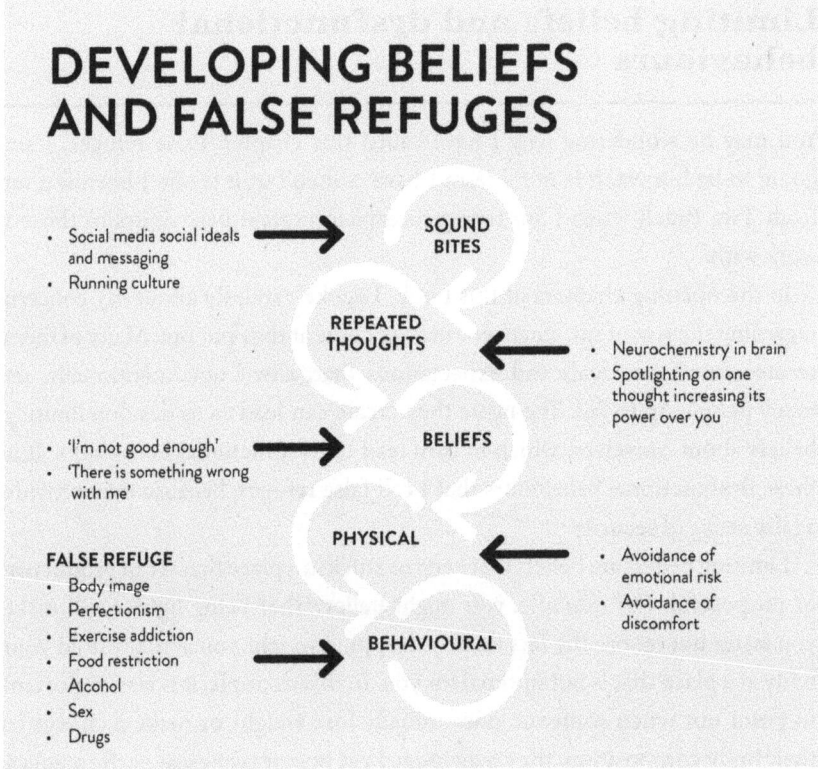

Figure 8.2

While I appreciate that it is a minefield to wade through all the (mis)information out there, one thing that can help is to be mindful of comparison. As the saying goes, comparison is the thief of joy. And in reality, the only person we can truly compare ourselves to is ourselves. At the same time, it is human nature to observe others and automatically make comparisons. So if we are going to do this, perhaps we should at least remind ourselves to make this a level playing field. We can definitely aspire to be professional athletes and be inspired by them, but it is important to appreciate that their lives are very different from ours. The structure of their lives rotates around performance and achieving because that is their job. And while a lot of us may fancy that career, we have to be realistic. Elite and professional athletes are outliers. Their body type, their physiology and their genetics are what make them adapt to training and progress at the level they do. Even if I dedicated my whole life to running, I would never go from my current marathon PB of 3:17 to a qualifying time to represent our country. I think it is fantastic when athletes appreciate their talent, have a healthy work ethic, surround themselves with appropriate support teams and meet their potential, but this is limited to a very small percentage of the population.

Run-fluencers are not athletes. They may not even be that talented, but perhaps they progress a little quicker because they don't have the constraints a lot of us have around work and home life. However, their lifestyles do generate envy and promise outcomes which I find dangerous and irresponsible.

On this note, let's take a minute to take stock and appreciate some actual facts which can help us to filter information and respond more appropriately, leading to a healthier and happier relationship with running (see Table 8.1).

RUN-FLUENCER LIFE	PRO ATHLETE LIFE	REALITY OF (MY) LIFE
Not paid to run but sometimes paid to create content. Often work time is also their training time. No real limitations, so they can create unrealistic ideals and expectations.	Paid to run but there is still structure around the day.	Full-time work that has little flexibility, so the available hours to run, train and recover are limited. Shift workers have further time considerations.
Work for multiple brands and adjust content to fit delivery rather than have a true alignment with and loyalty to a specific brand.	Genetically gifted and outliers.	Potentially have additional life stresses and pressures that add to overall load, increasing risk of injury and illness.
Create content to sell a product or event but often provide information based on solely their own experience, not qualifications.	Often contractually obliged to represent a brand that is providing sponsorship, or have athlete behaviours they have to adhere to if funded by a sporting body.	May work with a coach who can hold them accountable and ensure appropriate rest and recovery.
May hide behind a so-called professional title, e.g. 'I am a doctor and I run', but in reality they do very little hands-on professional work and their income comes from their content creation.	Usually target one or two A races a year, so have both an on-season and an off-season where they can rest and recover.	Need to consider financial implications for races, coaching, gym memberships and kit.
No race calendar as such and often do multiple races due to opportunity. Rarely schedule sufficient rest and recovery.	Usually have some form of support team around them, which may be hand-picked or allocated through their funding body.	

Table 8.1

Understanding dysfunctional behaviours

It is clear that societal messaging has a big part to play in how we value ourselves. Those of us who come from more complex backgrounds may be more influenced due to increased levels of self-doubt and low self-esteem. However, I think a lot of us, especially runners, tend to have personality traits that include an aspect of perfectionism. While there is definitely a spectrum to this, it is something that if not managed well can lead to dysfunctional thinking and then behaviours.

Something I observe a lot is the *'when* and *then'* mentality. That is, *when* I have (for example) a fast marathon time, *then* I will be successful. But will you? Will this be enough? The likelihood is that you will set another goal and then another. While there is no harm in having goals, it is important to become aware of your personality so you can learn ways to manage it.

All human behaviour serves a purpose, and this purpose is usually protection. Cast your mind back to being a young child and knowing you had done something wrong, like drawing on the walls. How many of you lied in an attempt to not get told off? While this is not life-threatening, it clearly demonstrates the innate bias we have to avoid suffering.

Dysfunctional behaviours such as disordered eating or exercise dependency equally serve a purpose of protection and often become a learnt coping mechanism when an individual feels like there is nowhere else to turn. These behaviours act as a method of denying emotions that are not only difficult to identify with but also don't want to be experienced. They often present themselves as feelings of discomfort and unease deep within, both physically and psychologically. We understand that something is not quite right; maybe life feels a bit messy or chaotic, but we can't quite articulate what is driving this. It is not always conscious; it is an experience almost like 'blind chatter' that fills us with a negative narrative fuelling a sense of unworthiness, which is fed by the information we have chosen to digest.

The act of achieving 'leanness' or 'being fit' or 'showing discipline' is a way of attaining something that we can't attain from our life. It is a means of proving our worth but becomes tied up in our identity, allowing us to create intrusive and catastrophic thinking which keeps us landlocked in negative beliefs about ourselves. These in turn drive our behaviours.

To quote Brené Brown, 'Perfectionism is a self destructive and addictive belief system that fuels this primary thought: if I look perfect, and do everything perfectly, I can avoid or minimise the painful feelings of shame, judgment, and blame.'

It's important to understand that it is your need to control all these uncomfortable thoughts and emotions that you project on to food, body image and running. It is much easier to work with areas of your life that you can control, contain and shape to help you 'feel okay'. However, as we discussed earlier, these behaviours provide a false sense of security and often become part of the overall problem, especially when they have negative consequences for your performance and, more importantly, your health.

Many of the individuals I work with are aware that their behaviours are not healthy or even serving them. However, these have become a familiar coping mechanism; humans are creatures of habit and we return to our familiar behaviours even when they may not be useful, as they somehow make us feel 'safe' in an uncertain world. When energy intake and levels are low, it can be even harder to challenge mindsets and create new, more helpful thought patterns. A malnourished body cannot feel happy, a malnourished body cannot feel content and a malnourished body cannot think clearly.

REDs and low energy availability

No book I write would be complete without a section on REDs. As one of the leading voices in this field, I understand this area and want to continue to educate people about it.

REDs, or relative energy deficiency in sport, is underpinned by low energy availability (LEA). That is, it occurs when there is not sufficient energy in the body to allow for the work that the individual wants to do. Work is defined as training but also includes daily movement and the energy cost of biological processes within the body, such as the brain, heart, lungs, and hormonal and digestive systems. However, while LEA underpins REDs, it is not the only factor – under-recovery, training stress and general life stress all contribute to this.

The human body has evolved to prioritise movement. This means that all energy consumed will first be used for physical activity. Energy availability is the amount of energy left over once energy for movement has been removed.

REDs is often associated with professional or elite-level athletes due to their high training loads, competitive environments and aspects of athlete mentality, which may lead to dysfunctional relationships with food and training. However, a recent study concluded that the incidence of LEA was around 19% in recreational female runners, so we can see that REDs and LEA are not restricted to the elite.[33] They can and do affect anyone who is physically active.

REDs is a condition that is multi-faceted. While LEA, possibly due to dysfunctional relationships with food, is one potential spoke, other key contributors include under-recovery both in day-to-day training and between races, and general stress on the nervous system.

Additionally, while LEA is problematic in both males and females, the female body is much more sensitive, so signs and symptoms tend to show up a lot quicker than in males. However, this is not to say that damage is not occurring when a male is in LEA; it just appears later. We know that studies are predominantly carried out on white males, which means that studies relating to ketogenic (low-carbohydrate) diets, fasting such as intermittent fasting or restrictive approaches don't show all of the potential negative consequences, especially when the study is over a short duration. If the same study was to be conducted over a longer period of two years, the likelihood is that the negative consequences associated with LEA would start to be demonstrated.

Types of REDs

There are two types of REDs – unintentional and intentional:

- **Unintentional or accidental REDs** is when the individual doesn't appreciate just how much energy is required to maintain biological function and training load. While they may present with similar symptoms to someone with intentional REDs, they are easy to work with as there is no psychological involvement, which means they are happy to implement nutritional and training interventions to get their body back to optimal.
- **Intentional REDs** is a conscious decision to restrict intake and/or overtrain. Technically, it involves some aspect of disordered eating and/or exercise dependency. When I am discussing this with individuals, they usually associate the start of these behaviours with the desire to change body composition – in most cases, to lose weight – because they have either been encouraged to do so by the culture within their sport or through comparison with fellow athletes, and they believe that this will improve their performance.

Symptoms of REDs

As I said earlier, the body will always prioritise movement. Just as your smartphone starts to shut down non-essential apps when it is running low on battery, your body does the same and down-regulates your metabolism to preserve energy. One thing to be mindful of is that REDs is not always associated with weight loss. You can have an individual who is in LEA at a normal or above-normal weight. The human body does not like being in huge energy deficits and this results in compensatory behaviours which can stop the body from losing weight. This is also why low-calorie diets do not work in the long term.

WARNING SIGNS

A number of key warning signs can be observed and these should not be ignored.

Physiological
- Lack of three consecutive periods in females or a change to a previously regular menstrual cycle
- Decline in morning erectile function in male athletes (less than five a week is a cause for concern)
- Changes to thermoregulation, and difficulties staying warm in the winter and cool in the summer months
- IBS-like symptoms due to gastroparesis (slow movement of food through the digestive system) and dysbiosis (a change in optimal microbiome)
- Changes to cardiac output
- Peripheral nerve damage[34]
- Potential autoimmune presentations such as Epstein–Barr virus (EBV) – see page 159

Performance
- Poor recovery between training sessions
- Recurrent injuries, including soft tissue, tendon and stress fractures
- Poor development of muscle mass and adaptation to training
- Increased risk and prevalence of infections and illness, making it difficult to train consistently

While the physiological and performance consequences are applicable to both types of REDs, the following symptoms are mainly associated with those who have intentional REDs.

Behavioural
- Preoccupation with and constantly talking about food
- Poor sleep patterns
- Restricting or strict control of food intake
- Overtraining or difficulties taking rest days
- Training through pain
- Ignoring advice regarding hormonal health restoration

Psychological
- Irrational behaviour
- Fear of food and weight restoration
- Severe anxiety
- Becoming withdrawn and reclusive
- An inability to decipher the difference between fact and intrusive thoughts and limiting beliefs

REDs recovery

While REDs is definitely becoming more mainstream, with many athletes from all walks of life discussing their experience, recovery is not simple or even linear.

I think this is probably my biggest concern – as with most things that are discussed publicly and based on a sample size of *n*=1, recovery from REDs is *not as simple as eating more and moving less*. So, what does recovery look like and how do you go about it?

Recovery involves biochemical, physiological and hormonal regulation. This takes time, but everyone's journey will be different. Contrary to what a lot of athletes portray on social media, no one recovers from REDs with a short-term period of rest or abstinence from sport. While this definitely helps, it is important to appreciate that REDs is fundamentally a metabolic injury and, like any injury, recovery is going to take time. Some research suggests a minimum of eighteen months for full recovery to occur and the body to be able to adapt from training again, but a lot of this also depends on the length of duration of the situation and the individual involved.

A good analogy is to think of your body as a bank account. When you are in REDs, you are way into your overdraft, in the red. A lot of people who acknowledge they have REDs understand that something needs to change, but find it hard to allow their body to return to a place where they can start to actually heal. So, just like an overdrawn bank account, you can save and get back to a bank balance of zero, but if you splash out on a holiday as soon as you get there, you will once again go into the red. In reality, we all have to learn to save up before we spend money on designer boots or fancy holidays, so that we can also continue to make our day-to-day payments without tipping back into our overdraft. The same applies to the human body.

Even once you get back to hormonal balance, you need to give your body sufficient time to store energy so that it can be directed to repair the full extent of the metabolic injury that extends beyond just hormones. This includes the production of red blood cells, healing the gut and digestive system, reversing damage to bone health and repairing grey and white matter in the brain to encourage the development of neural pathways involved in behaviour change; and then the body can finally start adapting to actual training both from a body composition and performance point of view.

Steps to recovery

1. Diagnosis by exclusion – if you suspect REDs, go and see a sports practitioner who is qualified and can read blood biomarkers and do a full clinical and behavioural assessment. It is unlikely that your GP will have much knowledge of REDs. That said, some do and many are keen to learn, which is why I have created a section later in this chapter about what medics should know about runners.
2. Those with intentional REDs – that is, whose behaviours around food and training are a conscious decision based on a belief – will not only need support with their physical health, but also psychological/behavioural input.
3. While not everyone needs to stop all training, it is likely that you will need to modify your training for the foreseeable future. It is a good idea to bring together those on your team who are involved in your training and care to discuss a realistic plan.
4. Consider adding activities that help to increase parasympathetic nervous system activity, such as mindfulness, drawing, knitting or yoga.
5. Appreciate that you will need to change your attitude and behaviours

going forward. You don't want to overcome REDs only to end up repeating the behaviours that got you there in the first place.

CASE STUDY

While a lot of people associate REDs with females, I wanted to showcase that it can impact males too. I want to thank Jake Smith, who has given me permission to discuss his case and was keen for me to put a name to his experience in order to help others.

Those of you who are in the road-running world will know that Jake is one of our promising marathon stars. In 2021 he was pace-making for the elite Cheshire Marathon when he decided to continue to the end, finishing in two hours and eleven minutes.

Jake approached me over eighteen months ago, following a right-sided sacral stress fracture, a DEXA (bone density) scan demonstrating osteoporosis in his lumbar spine and a diagnosis of REDs by his sports medicine consultant.

He presented with quite a complex history, especially his relationship with food and training. He was low in weight and had very low hormonal markers. However, he was also really motivated to engage in care and support his health in the primary instance and then get back to his performance. I explained to Jake that it was going to be a long recovery process and he needed to set some realistic goals with regard to races. He has a good relationship with his coach and over the last eighteen months I have worked with them both, as well as the extended sports medical team.

In the beginning, Jake found it very challenging to change his mindset about nutrition and training. He was used to his formula and found it hard to appreciate that the same behaviours which had worked so well for him in the first few years of his career had led to this outcome.

What I admire most about Jake is that, while the process was hard for him, he trusted the team around him. He started to understand how to listen to his body, and we have since had conversations where he has told me that he was pulling back a bit on training because he could sense that he was pushing harder than he needed to. I think this has been the biggest hurdle for him. Like most professional athletes, Jake has a real drive to achieve and this striving mentality is something he has had to really rein in at times.

The journey definitely has not been without its hiccups and bumps in the road, but it has been such a pleasure working with Jake and not just watching him return to his previous form but also observing his growth as an athlete. He now fuels well and rests sufficiently. Not only have his blood markers returned to normal, but he also appreciates that when he nurtures and nourishes his body, it responds and works for him.

Jake is a role model to other athletes. I would love to say that all my discussions with professional athletes in the same position lead to the same response and outcome, but sadly many athletes modify training and take on board advice only until their presenting symptoms have improved. They then return to the same behaviours and formulas, only to present with another injury, usually bone-related, within six months. Jake truly understood that everything needed to change if he was going to get his running career back on track again. He has given his body a real chance to recover and repair. He has worked on his mindset and he is not fearful of asking for help when he needs it. I am really excited to see how the next eighteen months pan out for him, and I am confident that he has a really bright future.

One last point on REDs...

One final point is for females who are on hormonal contraception. While tracking your hormonal health is one way of knowing if your body is working for you, this can be disguised if you are on hormonal contraception. Individuals on the combined oral contraceptive pill (COCP) may believe that they are having a regular cycle, but this is a withdrawal bleed, not an actual period. In fact, the COCP flatlines our hormonal health to prevent us from ovulating and becoming pregnant. This is also why it should no longer be the option of choice for women who have hypothalamic amenorrhoea (no periods for three months consecutively or when menses has not started under the age of sixteen). As it flatlines hormones and also contains a synthetic version of oestrogen, it has been shown to be contraindicated to support hormonal or bone health.

Similarly, the progesterone-only pill, hormonal IUD and implant all work on a mechanism to prevent pregnancy but often completely stop any form of bleeding.

So if you are a runner who may be worried about LEA and REDs but you are also on hormonal contraception, tracking your menstrual cycle is not going to be suitable for you. In these instances, I use a mix of blood tests, especially the thyroid hormone tests T4 and T3, which are directly linked to carbohydrate availability. Studies have shown that a low intake of carbohydrate for just a few days can decrease production of T3.[35] A prolonged low T3, also often associated with a low T4, will send messages to the hypothalamus to indicate that energy intake is too low, resulting in a down-regulation of all metabolic health, including the hormonal system. These tests in conjunction with assessing nutritional intakes, training load and general attitudes can give me a pretty good indicator of whether someone is in or at risk of LEA and thus REDs.

Looking after our hormonal health

Hormones are chemical messengers that are made by specialised cells within endocrine glands, and they are responsible for the correct function of the body.

When we think about hormones, for the majority of us, our thoughts turn to biology lessons and oestrogen and testosterone jump to mind. While these are indeed incredibly important for reproductive health and performance, they are two of a very long list. Others include insulin, growth hormone, leptin, ghrelin, cortisol, melatonin and the thyroid hormones T4 and T3, some of which we have already discussed. All of these have critical roles to play within our body, from maintaining metabolic function to ensuring progression and adaptation from our training, optimising bone health, appetite control and regulating sleep.

Regulating and maintaining our hormonal health, for both males and females, is central to our health and performance. Understanding how to harness the benefits of these amazing chemical messengers allows us to meet our potential.

Recap on energy availability

Modern society tends to encourage the message that we all need to move more and eat less. However, physiological studies have determined that the human body is biologically biased towards energy balance, so in reality we need to move more and eat more if we are to see the performance benefits from our training.

While there is a real emphasis on energy in versus energy out, this then ignores the importance of energy availability, which is 'the amount of energy available for biological function once the cost of movement has been subtracted from overall energy intake'. In other words, it is the energy left over to allow for all these chemical reactions to occur in our body.

While it has been a key theme throughout the book, it is clear to see how often the role of nutrition has been simplified. While one of its main roles is to ensure sufficient nutritional intake to allow the body to function and perform, this applies across all areas of our life, not just physical performance. Very few of us appear to be aware of the role nutrition plays at a cellular level and its involvement in the more intricate processes that need to occur in the body to allow optimal health and performance to occur.

As we described in the previous section about REDs and LEA, if we do not consume sufficient energy, in particular carbohydrate, to meet both these demands, then the body turns on compensatory behaviours that result in the down-regulation of metabolism and hormonal function. As we have seen, this has implications for our health and performance.

But how do these requirements and processes change as we move through our lifespan?

Adolescence

Adolescents have very high energy requirements, as they are also going through growth, development and puberty, all of which have a huge energy cost.

One of the key concerns with this age group is not meeting their energy requirements and delaying puberty. In females, if menstruation has not started by the age of sixteen, this is known as primary amenorrhoea and should not be ignored. Regardless of what you may hear, it is never okay for a female not to have a period without a valid medical reason.

Adolescence is the time when significant peak bone mass activity is occurring, but if there are disruptions to energy intake, growth and the onset of menstruation, this can have severe consequences.

Oestrogen in females and testosterone in males is the key component for optimal bone health, in addition to sufficient energy, calcium, and vitamins D and K. In those females where primary amenorrhoea occurs, they are at high risk of lower bone density and thus developing stress fractures. Similarly, males can disrupt puberty through restrictive eating and thus don't produce sufficient testosterone during those adolescent years. In fact, among some of the young runners I work with who are in their early twenties and have experienced hypogonadism (low oestrogen or testosterone), this appears to be the most likely time for them to develop their first stress fracture, and for some it is a long path of repeated injuries and inconsistent training. It is usually associated with a combination of training load and intensity increasing at this age, combined with a lower bone density. This is heightened further if the individual is still in LEA, as this disrupts bone turnover and replacement. Sadly, a statistic from 2010 reported that 54% of junior track and field medallists did not make it to senior level due to overtraining and overcompeting.[36]

The female factor

The menstruation years

While there is a lot of negative press about menstruation, it is important to appreciate that having a period is actually a good sign and a real barometer of health. It's basically saying that conditions are optimal for a pregnancy to occur. However, a period is more than just a reproductive portal. As we have already seen, delayed or no menstruation can have huge consequences on bone health and significantly increase the risk of injury. Additionally, oestrogen is really important for cognitive function, balance, proprioception, heart health, immune health and mood. With any reduction in oestrogen, there is a huge risk to overall health and performance (just ask any woman going through the perimenopause and menopause).

A normal menstrual cycle is defined as anything between twenty-three and thirty-five days. While textbooks generally discuss a twenty-eight-day cycle, very few women experience this. The key thing to be aware of is changes to your cycle, such as the cycle length getting longer or shorter, the flow getting lighter or heavier, the number of days of your cycle changing or your cycle stopping (secondary amenorrhoea), unless of course you have fallen pregnant.

Any deviation from your normal should not be ignored. There are many potential threats to our menstrual cycle. These can be medical or due to lifestyle, but regardless, all should be investigated.

Nutrition intake and nutrition timing, especially in women who are physically active, changes in body composition, and training load and volume can all interfere with your cycle, so tracking yours and being aware of change can help you to ensure that you are staying on top of your fuelling and training.

Contrary to what many women think, having a regular cycle also signifies that the rest of your hormones are most likely working in synergy. This includes growth hormone and testosterone, which are essential for laying down lean muscle mass and ensuring progression from training.

AN ODE TO CARBOHYDRATE

Recent studies by Danish researcher Anna Melin have confirmed that carbohydrate availability plays a key role in hormonal regulation and menstrual health, particularly in women who are physically active.

The rise in trends encouraging fasted training and avoiding carbohydrate have left a lot of women with irregular cycles or, in the worst cases, secondary amenorrhoea (the complete absence of cycles for three months or longer). And remember, no periods means no oestrogen, which impacts bone health and leaves you more susceptible to injury and also illness.

Contrary to what is claimed in the popular press, carbohydrates are not the enemy. In fact, I would go as far as saying they are essential for active women to stay healthy and to also allow for progression in their training and sport.

Recently, there has been a lot of noise around syncing your cycle to your running. What I want to point out here is that while we know there are potential trends, we definitely do not have the science to dictate that we should train in a particular way on a particular day of our cycle.

What we know is that in general women tend to feel more energised and less impacted by hormones in the follicular phase of their cycle, especially once menses has stopped. This also makes sense as the reproductive hormones involved are all quite low at this stage and there is little hormonal activity. However, once we move through ovulation and head into the luteal phase, there is a lot of hormonal activity, with both oestrogen and progesterone reaching their peaks and also declining during this time. It is these fluctuations in hormones that can cause disruption to our mood, temperature, appetite, energy levels and thus ability to train. This is why earlier in this book I mentioned the importance of increasing carbohydrate intake during the luteal phase of our cycle, as this can help to alleviate some of these potential issues.

However, I want to stress here that every single woman will experience their menstrual cycle differently. Some are totally unaffected, while others find they have absolutely no power to perform, especially in the days leading up to their period. Some women will experience more emotional symptoms, others more physical. There really is no absolute, which is why I get irritated and frustrated that female health is now becoming big business, with many brands and companies producing female-specific nutrition or products and cashing in with no clear evidence to back their claims.

The only real way to navigate your cycle is to track it and respond to your personal symptoms. If for example you always feel very low in energy in the three to five days before your period, then respect this and aim to do activity that feels more nurturing and supportive.

Some common trends that are worth taking into consideration include a higher body temperature during the luteal phase, which can impact sleep and thus recovery, so you may need to be mindful of this between harder training sessions. Similarly, a higher core temperature can impact your perceived exertion. This means that the same runs you did a week earlier might feel harder and slower. Work with these feelings, not your overall pace, as this helps to prevent injury risk. A higher core temperature can also mean higher fluid and sodium losses, so replace these, especially during runs and in hotter temperatures.

During the luteal phase when progesterone is dominant, a study in 2019 found that women perceived themselves as less attractive.[37] While this does not have a direct impact on running, it does demonstrate the power of hormones and how they can impact our thoughts and feelings too.

Perimenopause and beyond

Perimenopause or menopause transition begins several years prior to menopause. It usually starts in a woman's forties, but can start earlier in some cases and can last anything from a few months to ten years. Perimenopause stops at menopause, when the ovaries no longer produce any eggs and oestrogen levels are low.

Women will start to see declining levels of oestrogen from around the age of forty onwards. As we have previously discussed, oestrogen has several important functions relating to body composition, physical performance, bone health and cognitive function. In addition, oestrogen protects women from heart disease as it prevents the production of cholesterol. This is why the risk of heart disease increases in postmenopausal women.

It is very difficult to diagnose whether a woman is going through perimenopause. There are in the region of 200 potential symptoms which would indicate this, but we only tend to hear about the most common, such as hot flushes, fatigue, brain fog and joint pain. Lesser-known symptoms include digestive changes, low mood, changes to sport performance, dry eyes, dry skin, restless legs and heightened anxiety.

While it all does sound like doom and gloom, with advances in research and more women asking for information, there are a number of options that can help alleviate a lot of these symptoms and improve quality of life at this stage. As most of these symptoms are related to declining hormone levels, essentially oestrogen, HRT is highly recommended. While there has been a lot of negative press about HRT in the past, numerous options are available now, so it is definitely worth talking to your GP or hormonal health specialist to see if there is an approach that works best for you.

Personally, I have found this stage of life very challenging. Like most women, I had assumed I would know when I was in it, but the reality is that it's not as simple as that. In fact, I have described it as 'being in puberty but in reverse'!

Perimenopause is a time when hormones are constantly fluctuating. This is why every woman's experience will be so individual, but also why it is hard to tell what is going on from doing blood tests alone. The challenge is finding the right approach for you, and also appreciating that this may need to change as you transition through this phase of life.

While a lot of women experience more physical symptoms, I have mostly been impacted by difficult emotional symptoms, including very low mood at times, a huge loss in confidence and emotional dissociation. Contrary to what is often indicated, I still have a regular menstrual cycle and this is actually one of the reasons it took me a while to go and speak to my GP about my symptoms. For a while, I had just put them down to life stress. I am still working out what I need, but I am very fortunate that my GP here in Cumbria, Dr Cath Munro, is a specialist in menopause and also very open-minded and appreciative that women who are physically active often have different symptoms and needs from women with more sedentary lifestyles.

What I will say is that no one needs to suffer during this stage of life. My advice is to make sure you get the help you need, and that doesn't always mean HRT. Research has also shown that being and staying physically active can support your progression through perimenopause, often reducing the severity of a number of the symptoms associated with it. In particular, including more resistance training over cardio will not only help maintain lean muscle mass and thus body composition, but also prevent the natural decline in bone density often seen at this age.

From a dietary perspective, in general it has been found that following a Mediterranean-style diet best supports this phase of life. However, there should also be a focus on ensuring that there is enough protein in the diet to further prevent the usual decline in muscle mass associated in this population. Those who consume good amounts of protein have been shown to maintain 40% more muscle mass than those that have low intake of protein. The recommendations are 2–2.4 grams per kilogram of body weight daily.

During the perimenopause, bone health becomes a real concern; declining oestrogen levels reduce protection. Ensuring sufficient vitamin D and calcium, doing resistance training and using HRT can all help to prevent further loss.

SOCIETAL MISCONCEPTIONS

Many women who are going through perimenopause notice and struggle with changes to their body composition. Current misconceptions and Western societal beliefs mean that many women at this stage decide that the only way to combat this is through restrictive diets and removing carbohydrates.

Indeed, the latest research shows the complete opposite: declining oestrogen levels mean that the female body is no longer efficient at fat oxidation, which tends to spare our use of carbohydrates. Thus carbohydrate intakes, especially in those women who remain physically active, are critical not just for performance but also for counteracting the fatigue often associated with this phase of life. I tend to make recommendations based on activity level, but want to stress that no female, even those who are sedentary, should eat less than 3 grams of carbohydrate per kilogram of body weight per day.

Hormones are essential for life. We need them to perform physically and cognitively, but how many of us are actually aware of this? Ensuring sufficient energy and nutrient timing is key to allow the network of hormones within the human body to work optimally. For women, appreciating and understanding the power of their reproductive hormones, particularly oestrogen, and the many benefits to health and performance is empowering and definitely a conversation that needs to keep happening.

Exercise dependency

We all know exercise is good for us ... until it isn't.

While there is a lot of research on the merits of regular movement for our physical and mental health, there is also evidence that when exercise becomes something compulsive and starts to impact daily life, it actually becomes more of a problem to both physical and mental health.

The *Diagnostic and Statistical Manual of Mental Disorders* refers to exercise addiction as an excessive behavioural pattern or behavioural addiction.[38] While there are no specific diagnostic criteria based on this definition, the following symptoms are often used to indicate a dysfunctional relationship with exercise:

- persistent and intense exercising habits that lead to a physical and mental decline
- unsuccessful attempts to reduce the intensity or frequency of exercising
- irritability or other mood changes when not able to train or exercise
- recurrent preoccupation (persistent thoughts) related to exercise
- a tendency to lean on exercise to manage stress and other emotional states
- starting to have a negative impact on relationships and other areas of life due to exercise-related habits
- inability or difficulty reducing or stopping exercise despite negative experiences or consequences like sports injuries, muscular pain or illness
- hiding the frequency or intensity of exercise habits or events from others.

Fundamentally, if your relationship with running takes precedence over other areas of your life, or you notice increased distress, anxiety or irritability from not being able to run on a given day, this may suggest that running has become a maladaptive coping mechanism; or the term I prefer, a false refuge.

To a certain degree, I think most runners have slightly obsessive and compulsive personalities. I know I do, and I have admitted that there were definitely times, especially early on when I started running, when my relationship with running was unhealthy. I can see that I used it as a way of blocking out how I was feeling. Just as anorexia had numbed my feelings and needs as a teenager, running provided this as an adult. It is very common for one type of addiction or behavioural issue to morph into another, especially if the underlying difficulties have not been addressed. This is also why so many individuals who have previously experienced mental health issues or illness, or have been alcoholics or drug users, 'find running'. There is also some irony that the very behaviour that first supported mental health then becomes the behaviour that leads to a decline. Often these behaviours light up our reward centre in the brain, so is there any wonder we keep repeating them? But here is the crux: the more we use these behaviours to 'feel good', the harder we have to work within the behaviour to get our fix. I think this is why so many people move so quickly through ultra-long distances. What was initially enough doesn't quite hit the spot. As with most limiting beliefs and dysfunctional behaviours, it can be very hard to appreciate what is truly going on.

My relationship with running changed when I addressed the underlying thoughts and emotions. When it no longer became my way of attaining worth. I had created such an identity around it that I couldn't see that it was also my way of numbing all my insecurities. I realised I had a problem when I started noticing anxiety about not being able to run and I finally admitted to myself that I had a problem after trying to run while having a chest infection. I am not proud of this, but it was definitely my wake-up call.

I now have a much healthier relationship with running. I am aware that it would be easy for me to fall back into old behaviours, but I have learnt new, healthier strategies to cope with my insecurities, such as mindfulness, and have learnt not only to trust my body but also to listen to it. So even when Damian sets me a session, if I notice I am tired or I haven't been able to fuel appropriately due to work commitments, I will chat with him and we will change the plan. Sometimes this involves an extra rest day or two, and sometimes just a different type of run, but this way I get so much more enjoyment out of my running, and running really is something that brings me joy, social connection and a sense of community.

In the crazy world we live in, it can be easy to get caught up in 'more, more, more', but I want to stress that learning to listen to your body, nurture it and provide it with sufficient rest is always going to generate better results than using running as a way of escaping your problems.

It is also important to highlight here the link between exercise dependence and a higher risk of developing REDs. Something can seem like 'healthy' behaviour, but at the point when the individual is struggling to rest and/or limit this, it can lead to under-recovery, which as we know can contribute to REDs.

The most common causes for most of the running injuries I hear about with my clients are usually related to under-recovery and getting caught up in all the noise, always feeling like they will be happier when they have completed the next event ... and the next event and the next event.

If you feel like running has become more of an obsession and you can identify with some of the symptoms above, please do seek professional help. While the thought of changing your intensity and volume of running may create distress, in the long run it may actually benefit not just your running but your mental and physical health.

Body image

As you can probably tell by now, I find human behaviour fascinating. As I mentioned in earlier chapters, one of the biggest challenges in my work is individuals who believe that they need to have a certain body size or composition to be a good runner. In the majority of cases, these individuals try to maintain their body at a place that is too low for them. My words to them are always: 'suffering is not accepting reality'.

So when we choose to push back against our genetic predisposition, believing that we are not okay, fixating on our body image can be another false refuge.

The definition of body image is 'a person's emotional attitudes, beliefs and perceptions of their own body'. Many people project their insecurities on to their body because this is a lot easier to manage or change than dealing with the root of the problem. Often when we don't like who we are, this is what we perceive in our body. Many people punish and push their bodies in the belief that if they 'look the part' then everything will fall into place, but this is rarely the case – it is all a false promise.

It is of course natural to have some bad body image days. As we saw earlier, hormonal changes, particularly in women, can influence how we experience and view our body, but the issues come when the behaviours around trying to 'fix our body' become dysfunctional and extreme.

As a person of colour, I've always struggled with a sense of belonging, but this was heightened during my younger years. That said, to this day, I struggle to know when someone reacts badly towards me if that is a genuine dislike due to something I have said or if it is related to the colour of my skin. And while I have been successful in my life with regard to both running and work, this has definitely not come easy and I still have to overcome barriers to feel accepted, especially in the world of sport. However, this deep sense of not belonging, which I am now acutely aware of, was not something I totally understood when I was younger and it definitely played into my need to contain my body. As I explained earlier, part of my anorexia was a way of expressing how insignificant I felt in the world I was in.

For years I used to hear the narrative playing in my head: 'If you were just a bit thinner/leaner/taller, you would be more accepted by everyone. You would fit in.' Of course, I know now that this is not true. In fact, now I just feel so privileged to have the body I have and accept that it works for me. It allows me to have cool adventures in beautiful locations and, most importantly, it is the least interesting thing about me.

Overcoming issues with body image is hard, especially in a world where we objectify the body and there appears to be so much stigma around body fat. We have created so much scaremongering and it really saddens me because so many athletes, runners and individuals I work with don't meet their full athletic potential because they place so much value on how their body looks, rather than what it can do, especially when we nurture it.

What do medics need to know?

Before I wrote this section, I checked with a few of my friends who are medics to see if it would be useful to include. They all agreed that not only would it be beneficial for medics but also for the individual involved, as it gives them information they can take to their medical practitioner. While I will always advise individuals to see a medicinal practitioner if they have any concerns about their health, I have noticed that there can be a disparity in knowledge between what is appropriate for the general population and what is appropriate for someone who is physically very active, and on paper generally fit and healthy.

Ferritin

As we discussed earlier in the book, a ferritin store of less than 30 micrograms per litre would indicate iron deficiency. In general practice, the parameters are often lower, at 20 micrograms per litre; and for those of us who are even moderately active, running two or three times a week, we are definitely going to notice low ferritin stores. The recommendation for runners is ideally to have values above 50 micrograms per litre.

EBV

EBV (Epstein–Barr virus) is a very common virus that spreads easily and is best known for causing mononucleosis, or glandular fever. It has recently been associated with REDs. While the virus itself is highly contagious and may have been contracted in the past, it remains dormant in the body and can be reactivated. This is especially triggered by those who have a depressed immune system relating to low energy availability and/or under-recovery. I have seen this repeatedly in practice. Many runners do not give themselves enough time to recover, especially between ultra-distance events, while also training at a high intensity and combining this with other potential life stresses and demands. This results in a depressed immune system, which in turn switches on an autoimmune response and reactivates EBV.

It often presents as severe fatigue and has implications on physical performance, but there is no real quick fix. It can last as little as two weeks, or as long as three months or more if care is not taken to manage training load and overall stress. There is no real treatment for EBV, but it can be useful to do blood tests to identify if this is the cause and to help with overall management.

REDs versus perimenopause

As we have discussed previously, both of these conditions are usually associated with low hormonal levels, including oestrogen. Low energy availability down-regulates hormonal health and results in hypothalamic amenorrhoea, which is one potential presenting symptom of REDs. Equally, the perimenopause is a time when overall oestrogen levels are declining. Symptoms, especially those linked with low oestrogen levels, are similar, which means many women in their forties are often diagnosed with perimenopause when indeed they are actually in low energy availability.

Why does this matter? You could argue it doesn't, as the likelihood is that once a woman has reached this stage of life, the chances of wanting any (further) children are low and so treating for perimenopause with HRT is not going to do any harm. However, it can mean that REDs and LEA go undiagnosed. So, while the addition of HRT may help some symptoms, it is unlikely that overall performance will improve until the LEA is also addressed.

CASE STUDY

Last year I worked with a lady in her early fifties. She was a keen and very good trail runner and spent a lot of her time running in the mountains. She presented with a decline in performance, a loss of motivation and general fatigue. She had been to see her GP, who had rightly diagnosed perimenopause and had started her on HRT. However, twelve months later, she still wasn't feeling much better, which is why she had booked in with me.

When I checked her bloods, it was clear she had some definite signs of LEA – her T4 and T3 were both low, suggesting low carbohydrate availability. She also had low ferritin levels, which is another potential symptom of LEA due to lack of energy to make red blood cells.

On assessment of her nutritional intake, it was clear that she had been avoiding carbohydrates because of the concerns around changes to her body composition associated with perimenopause.

We had a long discussion about the importance of carbohydrates, especially at this stage of life and especially as she was so active. I also encouraged her to swap a couple of runs for resistance training. We increased her carbohydrate and protein intake. Three months later, she contacted me and said she had been feeling much better and her body composition had improved.

PCO versus PCOS

This is a really important and common mistake I see a lot in clinic. Many women are diagnosed with PCOS (polycystic ovary syndrome) when they have PCO (polycystic ovaries).

PCO is quite common – if you did an ultrasound on most women, you would see multiple follicles on the ovaries. It is particularly common in women who have had hypothalamic amenorrhoea (HA) and are trying to restore their hormonal health, but haven't quite got all the pieces of the puzzle to turn menstruation on.

HA is the condition associated with not having menstruation. It is known as primary if menses has not begun by the time a female is sixteen years old, and secondary when a female has previously had a menstrual cycle but this has stopped for three months or more. The most common cause of HA is lifestyle behaviours associated with restrictive eating, weight changes and exercise load. Contrary to what is often thought, you don't have to be underweight to have low energy availability and you don't have to be underweight to have HA, which is where a lot of the confusion comes in. Women who are a normal weight without a menstrual cycle may show multiple follicles on an ultrasound, and they are often misdiagnosed as having PCOS due to their physical appearance rather than looking at all the facts and individual history or behaviours.

PCOS is a metabolic condition that affects a lot of women but needs to be diagnosed by the Rotterdam criteria, which clearly state that an individual should have two of the following symptoms:[39]

- Ovulatory dysfunction in the absence of any other potential cause. This is the key point and is often overlooked by a lot of medics, especially when the individual presents looking 'healthy' because they are a normal weight and/or participate in regular exercise. The main takeaway here is that a recent history of, or ongoing recovery from, restrictive eating and/or excessive exercise (even if these have both been modified in recent months) can contribute to menstrual dysfunction and must be taken into consideration before diagnosing PCOS.
- Clinical or physical signs of hyperandrogenism, such as hirsutism, acne or elevated levels of total or free testosterone.
- Multiple follicles on an ultrasound, defined as a follicle number per ovary of twenty or more in at least one ovary.
- Thick uterine lining (in contrast to HA, where there is a thin uterine lining) on an ultrasound.

COCP versus HRT

As I have discussed, one of the key concerns in women with HA is around the implications this has for bone health. If HA is prolonged, it can cause an increase in the occurrence of stress fractures, which is not ideal for anyone but definitely not for a woman who runs.

Many young women in particular who present with one or more stress fractures as a result of HA and a DEXA which shows low bone density should be provided with medical care to support their bone health and prevent any further decline. The International Olympic Committee and British Menopause Society recommend the use of transdermal HRT and not the combined oral contraceptive pill (COCP) that so many medics put women on. The COCP is a contraceptive and thus down-regulates hormonal health. It does not 'reboot' it. Additionally, it has been shown that the synthetic oestrogen in COCP is contraindicated for bone health and can actually cause worsening symptoms, especially in the presence of LEA.

Current guidelines recommend HRT in conjunction with supporting hormonal health through restoration of energy availability and modification of exercise behaviours.[40]

What's wrong with me?

I am very aware that there is a lot of information in this section. I wanted to create a simple summary so that you can try and work out what may be going on for you and fast-track to the support and advice you need.

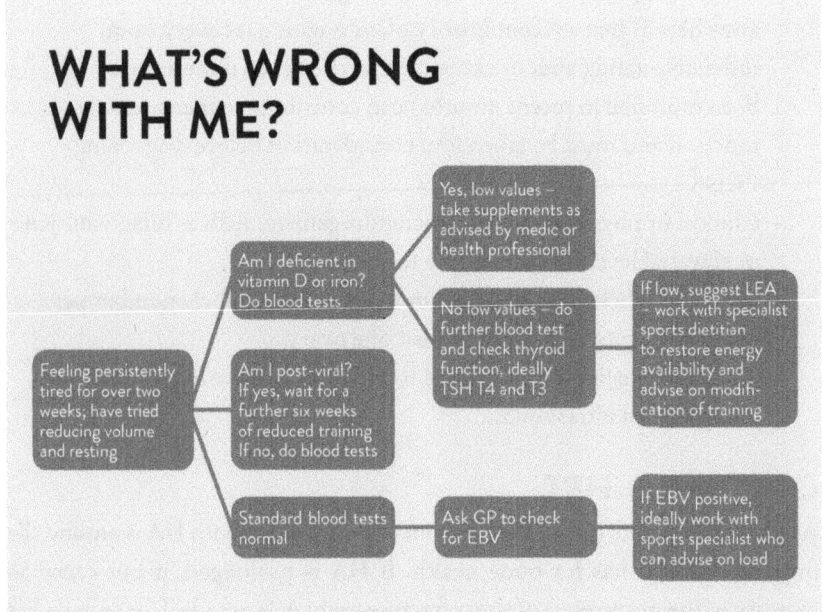

Figure 8.3

Unhealthy behaviours are not always visible. If you suspect LEA and REDs, it can be worth asking yourself the following questions:
- Do I find it difficult to have complete rest days?
- Have I had recurrent ligament or tissue damage in the last twelve months?

- Have I had a stress fracture in the last twelve months?
- (For males), do I have fewer than five morning erections per week?
- (For females), have my periods become lighter, become more erratic or stopped completely?
- Do I get anxious eating food away from home or that I have not prepared?
- Do I avoid social situations due to anxiety around food?
- Does my body weight/image impact my mood and ability to accept myself?
- Do I feel the need to exercise daily to justify eating?
- Have I noticed feelings of worsening low mood, irrational thoughts and increased anxiety?

If you answer yes to two or more of these questions, seek appropriate support.

DOS AND DON'TS

DON'T	DO
If you currently do not have a menstrual cycle, **don't** run.	**Do** go and see your GP/sports specialist and get appropriate advice.
If you have had more than one stress fracture and have been diagnosed with low bone density on DEXA, **don't** accept COCP as treatment in females or testosterone in males.	**Do** push for HRT in women and work with a sports dietitian to restore energy availability and support bone health.
If you are experiencing pain or discomfort when running which you can score as more than three out of ten, **don't** continue to run.	**Do** see a physio and get professional support.
Don't get caught up with comparison or peer pressure with regard to running volume, races or race distance.	**Do** what feels intuitively right for you and use the guidance in this book to help ascertain where you are in your running journey and what is appropriate with regards to next steps.
Don't get your nutrition and coaching advice from a popular celebrity or run-fluencer.	**Do** seek appropriate advice from qualified professionals; ensure that they not only have the right credentials but have also worked hands-on in the field of play.
Don't ignore changes to mood, motivation to run, sleep patterns or changes to your hormonal health.	**Do** track these symptoms and talk to your GP in the first instance, but be prepared to work with a sports specialist.
If you feel you *should* run rather than *want* to run, **don't**.	**Do** run for social connection, benefitting from being outside and general well-being (as long as you are not too tired or injured).
Don't succumb to trends and fads – they usually involve a false promise and someone trying to sell you something.	**Do** learn to listen to your body, nurture it and respect it for consistency and enjoyment.
Don't avoid carbohydrates.	**Do** include good sources of carbohydrates throughout the day, especially around training sessions.

FUEL FOR THOUGHT

DON'T	DO
Don't give protein a halo effect.	**Do** include protein as a response to exercise and increase your intake as you get older for both males and females. Consider using this as a source of fuelling in long endurance events to reduce muscle breakdown.
Don't avoid fats, especially unsaturated versions.	**Do** include unsaturated fatty acids, especially omega-3 fatty acids, and remember that the fatty acids in dairy are an exception to the saturated fat rule.
Don't displace macronutrients with fruits and vegetables.	**Do** include regular helpings of fruit, vegetables, wholegrains and beans to support your gut microbiome.
Don't reduce the human body to calories in versus calories out.	**Do** learn to listen to your internal cues and respond to your body and appetite.
Don't fixate on weight over performance.	**Do** provide your body with appropriate nutrition around your running and training schedule and let your body composition arrive at the place where it is optimal for you.

CHAPTER 9

Running for life

The aim of this book is to educate and inform with practical advice and solutions so that you can navigate the noise around running. It is also an opportunity to share my experiences, both personally and professionally, to not only demonstrate what I have learnt over many years of working in sport and with athletes, but to show you that I too am a runner, I too have been distracted by the noise and I too have not always had a healthy relationship with running.

That said, running and my work have both shown me the importance of belonging, contributing and community; while being a person of colour in both these areas has definitely not been straightforward. In my work, I have dealt with many barriers related to the colour of my skin, but I have also been handed opportunities which have showcased my expertise, providing evidence that I am very good at what I do and confidence to believe this fact.

Similarly, in running, while I am always in the minority, and often even to this day the only person of colour at the start of a race, I have put aside my feelings of discomfort and forged ahead in an attempt to be a role model for others and push the narrative. You can't be what you don't see!

I'm hugely grateful to communities like Black Trail Runners, Black Girls Do Run, Muslim Runners and Muslim Hikers and Opening Up The Outdoors, who are changing the lie of the land and encouraging more people from minority groups to participate in activities in the great outdoors.

Amongst all the advice and practical suggestions, you have probably picked up that my own relationship with food, my body and running has taken many twists and turns. I have learnt many lessons and, while my dysfunctional relationships have been behind me for many decades, the experience still helps me today to engage, emphasise, support and provide hope that we can change our story and also our path to live a freer, more colourful life.

So, for anyone who needs to hear it today, a final instalment of my story, which I hope brings a smile and hope …

As I sat on the windowsill of my year 10 classroom, I could feel the warmth of the sun on my back. I was desperate for this heat. It was May and the temperature outside was typical of the month – mild, cloudy, but with sunny outbreaks. I could hear the laughter from outside, teenage girls in little clusters scattered all over the courtyard, deep in animated conversations. From within the classroom, there was also chatter: conversations about lunch, who was dating who and plans for the weekend. I tried to focus on what was being discussed, a smile painted on my face, trying to demonstrate that I actually cared; when in reality all I could focus on was willing the sun to warm up my shivering body, which was buried beneath layers of clothing. While everyone else was in full summer uniform of striped blue and white blouse and navy skirt, I was still sporting full thermals topped with a jumper and blazer to cover my tiny, vulnerable, undernourished body.

Unless you have experienced a restrictive eating disorder like anorexia, you will not truly be able to appreciate or understand the cold. Even in the height of summer, it seeps into every corner of you, deep into your bones, to the point where it aches to move. I don't remember much of this time, but I will never forget what it felt like to be so cold I was numb; to feel so incredibly alone, enhanced by the sheer void and emptiness that had been created within me. There is an extreme isolation that envelops you, repelling any form of care, love or comfort, and at the same time also shields you from further hurt, pain and suffering. It takes you to a place where thoughts are dark and intrusive but also loud. *You are not good enough. Nobody likes you.* The more isolated you become, the more these thoughts become dominant and become your truth.

My recovery from anorexia was not linear; it never is. Indeed, it has taken me over two decades to appreciate this and understand that even at times when I thought I had 'recovered', where food really was no longer an issue, there was still a problem. It has only really been in the last ten years that I have been able to see that the discomfort, lack of belonging and insignificance I felt at the age of thirteen and denied through restrictive eating has plagued me through my adult life. I just used other methods to try and fix it.

I spent my twenties worrying too much; always chasing something – the perfect job, the number on the scale, collecting accolade after accolade to prove I was enough, always in search of that ultimate pair of skinny jeans that worked for me.

In my thirties, I chased run paces and finishing times at races. I beat myself up daily for not being an earth mother, feeling a continual disappointment as a wife and never feeling satisfied with my career path. The search for the perfect pair of jeans continued.

In my forties, I've faced more losses, hurt and adversity, but finally I have stopped chasing. I have found acceptance and belief. I stopped and took stock. The answers were always there, within me; I just needed to understand. That is, I just needed to understand me.

I have come to the realisation that there has always been so much evidence that I'm enough just the way I am but I chose not to see it; there was always love and friendship that I denied myself because I didn't feel worthy.

I've stopped chasing happiness because it's not a destination, it's not a body aesthetic, it's not about having a partner; it's not about being successful or receiving external validation through work or races. It is a place you reach when you learn to forgive yourself and embrace being uniquely you. It is a place where you can sit comfortably in your skin, being grateful for those who bring love and laughter into your life; where you can drink coffee and eat cake without care; where you don't assume that acceptance and approval is based on what you look like. It is where you do what makes you smile, whether that's a run in the mountains or dancing in the kitchen, and it's not about creating an illusion of the 'type' of person you want the world to think you are.

It's about being true to yourself and maintaining authenticity, even when the chips are down.

Love,
R x

REFERENCES

1. Colak, M., Bingol, O.S. & Dayi, A. (2023). 'Self-esteem and social media addiction level in adolescents: The mediating role of body image'. *Indian Journal of Psychiatry*, 65(5), 595–600. https://doi.org/10.4103/indianjpsychiatry.indianjpsychiatry_306_22

2. Semenova, E.A., Fuku, N. & Ahmetov, I.I. (2019). 'Chapter Four - Genetic profile of elite endurance athletes'. In Barh, D. & Ahmetov, I.I., *Sports, Exercise, and Nutritional Genomics*, Academic Press, 73–104. https://doi.org/10.1016/B978-0-12-816193-7.00004-X

3. Science Training (23 April 2021). 'How does stress impact long-distance runners?' https://www.sciencetraining.io/2021/how-does-stress-impact-long-distance-runners/ accessed 5 November 2024.

4. Champion Sports Performance. 'Consistency: The overlooked key to help athletes reach their potential, stay injury-free and separate themselves from the crowd', https://www.championsp.com/consistency-the-overlooked-key-to-help-athletes-reach-their-potential/#:~:text=The%20athletes%20who%20train%20most,with%20lower%20risk%20of%20injury accessed 5 November 2024.

5. Jäger, R., Mohr, A.E., Carpenter, K.C. et al. (2019). 'International Society of Sports Nutrition position stand: Probiotics'. *Journal of the International Society of Sports Nutrition*, 16(1), 62. https://doi.org/10.1186/s12970-019-0329-0

6. World Health Organization fact sheet (1 March 2024). 'Obesity and overweight', https://www.who.int/news-room/fact-sheets/detail/obesity-and-overweight accessed 5 November 2024.

7. Shah, V.N, DuBose, S.N, Li, Z. et al. (2019). 'Continuous glucose monitoring profiles in healthy nondiabetic participants: A multicenter prospective study'. The Journal of Clinical Endocrinology & Metabolism, 104(10), 4356–4364. https://doi.org/10.1210/jc.2018-02763

8. Cox, C.E. (2017). 'Role of physical activity for weight loss and weight maintenance'. *Diabetes Spectrum*, 30(3), 157–160. https://doi.org/10.2337/ds17-0013

9. Fensham, N.C., Heikura, I.A., McKay, A.K.A. et al. (2022). 'Short-term carbohydrate restriction impairs bone formation at rest and during prolonged exercise to a greater degree than low energy availability'. *Journal of Bone and Mineral Research*, 37(10), 1915–1925. https://doi.org/10.1002/jbmr.4658

10. Donini, L.M., Barrada, J.R., Barthels, F. et al. (2022). 'A consensus document on definition and diagnostic criteria for orthorexia nervosa.' *Eating and Weight Disorders*, 27, 3695–3711. https://doi.org/10.1007/s40519-022-01512-5

11. Allen, N., Kelly, S., Lanfear, M. et al. (2024). 'Relative energy deficiency in dance (RED-D): A consensus method approach to REDs in dance.' *BMJ Open Sport & Exercise Medicine*; 10:e001858. https://doi.org/10.1136/bmjsem-2023-001858

12 Fensham, N.C., Heikura, I.A., McKay, A.K.A. et al. (2022). 'Short-term carbohydrate restriction impairs bone formation at rest and during prolonged exercise to a greater degree than low energy availability'. *Journal of Bone and Mineral Research*, 37(10), 1915–1925. https://doi.org/10.1002/jbmr.4658

13 Tiller, N.B., Roberts, J.D., Beasley, L. et al. (2019). 'International Society of Sports Nutrition position stand: Nutritional considerations for single-stage ultra-marathon training and racing'. *Journal of the International Society of Sports Nutrition*, 16, 50. https://doi.org/10.1186/s12970-019-0312-9

14 Tiller et al., 'International Society of Sports Nutrition position stand: Nutritional considerations for single-stage ultra-marathon training and racing'.

15 Sims, S.T., Mackay, K., Leabeater, A. et al. (2022). 'High prevalence of iron deficiency exhibited in internationally competitive, non-professional female endurance athletes—a case study'. *International Journal of Environmental Research and Public Health*, 19(24), 16606. https://doi.org/10.3390/ijerph192416606

16 Yang, J., Li, Q., Feng, Y. & Zeng, Y. (2023). 'Iron deficiency and iron deficiency anemia: Potential risk factors in bone loss'. *International Journal of Molecular Sciences*, 24(8), 6891. https://doi.org/10.3390/ijms24086891

17 Wiertsema, S.P., van Bergenhenegouwen. J., Garssen J. & Knippels, L.M.J. (2021). 'The interplay between the gut microbiome and the immune system in the context of infectious diseases throughout life and the role of nutrition in optimizing treatment strategies'. *Nutrients*, 13(3), 886. https://doi.org/10.3390/nu13030886

18 Mach, N. & Fuster-Botella, D. (2017). 'Endurance exercise and gut microbiota: A review.' *Journal of Sport and Health Science*, 6(2), 179–197. https://doi.org/10.1016/j.jshs.2016.05.001

19 Guest, N.S., Van Dusseldorp, T.A., Nelson, M.T. et al. (2021). 'International Society of Sports Nutrition position stand: Caffeine and exercise performance'. *Journal of the International Society of Sports Nutrition*, 18(1). https://doi.org/10.1186/s12970-020-00383-4

20 Baar, K. (2017). 'Minimizing injury and maximizing return to play: Lessons from engineered ligaments'. *Sports Medicine*, 47 (Suppl. 1), 5–11. https://doi.org/10.1007/s40279-017-0719-x

21 König, D., Oesser, S., Scharla, S. et al. (2018). 'Specific collagen peptides improve bone mineral density and bone markers in postmenopausal women—a randomized controlled study'. *Nutrients*, 10(1), 97. https://doi.org/10.3390/nu10010097

22 Zdzieblik, D., Oesser, S. & König, D. (2021). 'Specific bioactive collagen peptides in osteopenia and osteoporosis: Long-term observation in postmenopausal women'. *Journal of Bone Metabolism*, 28(3), 207–213. https://doi.org/10.11005/jbm.2021.28.3.207

23 Mendoza, K, Smith-Warner, S.A., Rossato, S.L. et al. (2024). 'Ultra-processed foods and cardiovascular disease: Analysis of three large US prospective cohorts and a systematic review and meta-analysis of prospective cohort studies'. *The Lancet Regional Health – Americas*, 37, 100859, https://doi.org/10.1016/j.lana.2024.100859

24 James, L.J., Stevenson, E.J., Rumbold, P.L.S. & Hulston, C.J. (2019). 'Cow's milk as a post-exercise recovery drink: Implications for performance and health'. *European Journal of Sport Science*, 19(1), 40–48. https://doi.org/10.1080/17461391.2018.1534989

25 ScienceDaily (11 April 2019). 'Eggs for breakfast benefits those with diabetes', University of British Columbia Okanagan campus. https://www.sciencedaily.com/releases/2019/04/190411101835.htm accessed 5 November 2024.

26 Murray, B. & Rosenbloom, C. (2018). 'Fundamentals of glycogen metabolism for coaches and athletes'. *Nutrition Reviews*, 76(4), 243–259. https://doi.org/10.1093/nutrit/nuy001

27 McCleery, J., Diamond, E., Kelly, R., et al. (2024). 'Centering the female athlete voice in a sports science research agenda: A modified Delphi survey with Team USA athletes'. *British Journal of Sports Medicine* 2024; 58:1107–1114. https://bjsm.bmj.com/content/58/19/1107

28 Rogan, M.M. & Black, K.E. (2023). 'Dietary energy intake across the menstrual cycle: A narrative review'. *Nutrition Reviews*, 81(7), 869–886. https://doi.org/10.1093/nutrit/nuac094

29 Silva, T.R., Oppermann, K., Reis, F.M. & Spritzer, P.M. (2021). 'Nutrition in menopausal women: A narrative review'. *Nutrients*, 13(7), 2149. https://doi.org/10.3390/nu13072149

30 Mata, F., Valenzuela, P.L., Gimenez, J. et al. (2019). 'Carbohydrate availability and physical performance: Physiological overview and practical recommendations'. *Nutrients*, 11(5), 1084. https://doi.org/10.3390/nu11051084

31 Murray, B. & Rosenbloom, C. (2018). 'Fundamentals of glycogen metabolism for coaches and athletes'. *Nutrition Reviews*, 76(4), 243–259. https://doi.org/10.1093/nutrit/nuy001

32 Reddy, S., Reddy, V. & Sharma, S. (2024). 'Physiology, circadian rhythm' [Updated 2023 May 1]. In: *StatPearls [Internet]. Treasure Island (FL): StatPearls Publishing*; 2024 Jan. Available from: https://www.ncbi.nlm.nih.gov/books/NBK519507/

33 Karlsson, E., Alricsson, M. & Melin, A. (2023). 'Symptoms of eating disorders and low energy availability in recreational active female runners'. *BMJ Open Sport & Exercise Medicine* 2023;9. https://doi.org/10.1136/bmjsem-2023-001623

34 Teixeira, A.L., Junho, B.T., Barros, J.L. & Gomez, R.S. (2016). 'Anorexia nervosa presenting as a subacute sensory-motor axonal polyneuropathy'. *Brazilian Journal of Psychiatry*, 38(2), 180. https://doi.org/10.1590/1516-4446-2015-1846

35 *British Journal of Sports Medicine* blog (14 August 2023). 'A bad situation made worse: Low carbohydrate intake amplifies low energy availability hormonal disturbances'. https://blogs.bmj.com/bjsm/2023/08/14/a-bad-situation-made-worse-low-carbohydrate-intake-amplifies-low-energy-availability-hormonal-disturbances/ accessed 5 November 2024.

36 Hollings, S. & Hume, P. (2010). 'Is success at the World Junior Athletics Championships a prerequisite for success at World Senior Championships or Olympic Games? – Prospective and retrospective analyses'. *New Studies in Athletics* 25. 65–77.

37 Krohmer, K., Derntl, B. & Svaldi, J. (2019). 'Hormones matter? Association of the menstrual cycle with selective attention for liked and disliked body parts'. *Frontiers in Psychology*, 10, 851. https://doi.org/10.3389/fpsyg.2019.00851

38 *Diagnostic and Statistical Manual of Mental Disorders* (2022), fifth edition, text revision DSM-5-TR.

39 Nicky Keay (2024), *Hormones, Health and Human Potential*.

40 Keay, *Hormones, Health and Human Potential*.

ACKNOWLEDGEMENTS

I want to say a huge thank you to Vertebrate, especially to Kirsty Reade for once again believing in me and encouraging me to write a book that we know will help and inform so many, and also to share a little more about me, Renee, the sports dietitian, the author, the runner.

As always, I want to thank all my friends who have supported me from near and far while I sat at home day after day writing this book. Thanks to those of you who made yourself available to run with me when I needed a break. And especially to Ellie Green, who kept my spirits high with her almost daily voice notes which always brought a smile to my face.

A huge thank you also to the athletes and individuals I have spoken to in order to provide a bit more context about some of the topics, in particular Damian Hall, Elsey Davis, Germain Grangier, Jake Smith, Kirsty Reade, Shane Ohly and Matt Hickman. And thanks also to Tim Halsey and Debbie Martin-Consani for reading the book before publication.

A big thank you to Jenny Tough for being an amazing inspiration but also someone I am lucky enough to call my friend and for agreeing to write the foreword.

Finally, a huge thanks to Ewen, my girls Maya and Ella, and my boys Bailey and Bosco, for allowing life to continue even when I was sleeping and breathing this book, and for the endless cups of tea and biscuits that help to fuel my brain.

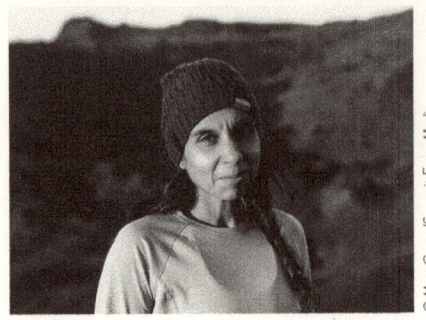

ABOUT THE AUTHOR

Renee McGregor is a leading sports and eating disorder specialist dietitian with over twenty years' experience working in clinical and performance nutrition. She has worked with athletes across the globe at Olympic level (Rio 2016) and has provided team management on numerous occasions at major championships in a variety of sports. She is the nutrition lead for English and Scottish National Ballet and was actively involved in producing the consensus statement about the management of REDs in dance. She is one of the leading voices in the country in REDs, female hormonal health and performance nutrition, and works with a number of professional athletes, teams and brands on a consultancy basis providing expert support on REDs and ensuring nutritional and clinical guidance for both performance and health. Renee is the bestselling author of *More Fuel You, Training Food, Fast Fuel* and *Orthorexia: When Healthy Eating Goes Bad*, and she writes a monthly column for Runner's World. She is often asked to comment and provide technical support for news and media, and she was the clinical advisor for the BBC documentary *Freddie Flintoff: Living with Bulimia*. Renee is a Montane athlete and a trustee for Black Trail Runners, supporting and advocating the importance of increased diversity and accessibility to minority groups to the outdoors. When not inspiring others with her work, Renee can be found running in the mountains and chasing the trails around her home in the Lake District. In 2022, she became British trail running champion for the short distance in her age group and finished third female in the Montane Summer Spine Sprint. In 2023, she finished fourth female and within the top ten in the Mustang Trail Race in Nepal.